Health, Disease and Medicine in Canada

A Sociological Perspective

Barry Edginton, Ph.D.

Professor
University of Winnipeg

Butterworths
Toronto and Vancouver

The Butterworth Group of Companies

Canada	Butterworths Canada Ltd., 2265 Midland Ave., TORONTO, Ont., M1P 4S1 and 409 Granville St., Ste. 1455 VANCOUVER, B.C., V6C 1T2
Australia	Butterworths Pty Ltd., SYDNEY, MELBOURNE, BRISBANE, ADELAIDE, PERTH, CANBERRA AND HOBART
Ireland	Butterworth (Ireland) Ltd., DUBLIN
Malaysia	Malayan Law Journal Sdn Bhd., KUALA LUMPUR
New Zealand	Butterworths of New Zealand Ltd., WELLINGTON and AUCKLAND
Singapore	Butterworth & Co (Asia) Pte Ltd., SINGAPORE
United Kingdom	Butterworth & Co (Publishers) Ltd., LONDON and EDINBURGH
USA	Butterworth Legal Publishers, ST PAUL, Minnesota, SEATTLE, Washington, BOSTON, Massachusetts, AUSTIN, Texas and D & S Publishers, CLEARWATER, Florida

Canadian Cataloguing in Publication Data

Edginton, Barry
  Health, disease and medicine in Canada

Bibliography: p.
Includes index.
ISBN 0-409-80530-0

1. Social medicine – Canada. I. Title.

RA418.3.C2E33 1989   362.1'0971   C89-093267-0

Sponsoring Editor: Gloria Vitale
Freelance Projects Coordinator: Joan Chaplin
Editor: Kathleen Hamilton
Cover Design: Joan Chaplin
Production: Jim Shepherd

Introduction

There are many different reasons for taking a medical sociology course. Sociology students may see the study of medical sociology as a way of understanding some of the larger social issues and their relation to the health-care system, as well as a way of dealing with their personal experiences and fears. Other students may have an interest in alternative forms of medical care since their faith in current medical practice has been eroded by the potentially harmful effects of drugs and medical technology. There are also concerns about the gender[1] and cultural biases of the health-care system, and a criticism of the current ways of defining who is sick and who is well (Turner 1987).

Ideas about health, illness and medicine are as varied as the reasons students give for taking a medical sociology course. Each one of us, however, has a specific model of health that is based on our experiences. More often than not, we tend to accept current scientific and medical explanations of health and health care. Today there is a trend toward looking to science for explanations of behaviour, and this makes us want sociology to act like a natural science, which it is not (Giddens 1982:2).

Students new to the sociological approach may be drawn to the study of medical sociology because of the popularity of health and the link between medicine and science. These students may have little faith in, or understanding of, sociology. They may think that sociology has little to offer since the social sciences are not "hard" or "real," as are the natural sciences.

Medicine and sociology are separate disciplines with different assumptions, goals and methods of inquiry. Each has its own way of viewing health and uses its own specific terminology to discuss and analyze health. Sociology and medicine *should* not have a common approach.

Whatever the reasons for the interest in medical sociology, students should start with an open mind and see all that sociology can offer in understanding health and the practice of medicine. The intention of this text is to answer some current questions, while developing new questions to apply to future developments in health care.

In Canada, sociology as an academic discipline is a "post World War II phenomenon; a substantive role for the sociology of health only developed during the past decade [1966-1976]" (Badgley 1976,3). Badgley (1976,3) goes on to say that the development of research in Canada has been shaped by the institutions which have sought the assistance of medical sociologists. For example, many of the articles presented in the first report on "The Sociology of Health in Canada" in *Social Science and Medicine* (1976, vol. 10, no. 1) were written by researchers working in medical or paramedical institutions. With the expansion of medical sociology over the past decade and the growth of opportunities for medical sociologists in academic institutions, medical schools and government departments, the questions for research and the scope of the field have expanded considerably to include a larger definition of the field (Kelner and New 1984,189). The second issue on Canadian research in *Social Science and Medicine*, which appeared in 1984, did little to expand the scope of the field, and failed to address many of the current issues in Canadian health care. However, new material is slowly appearing. There are now readers in the sociology of medicine: *Health and Canadian Society* (Coburn et al. 1987) and *Sociology of Health Care in Canada* (Bolaria and Dickinson 1988). There is also a work on sociological issues in medical care: *The Canadian Health Care System* (Crichton, Lawrence and Lee 1984). These books show a need for the development of the field of medical sociology in Canada. They also indicate how the separation of sociological work done inside and outside the medical system is dictated by the institutional setting of the researcher (Evans 1984,289).

This text is critical of our present health-care system and the medial profession. Without following any specific sociological model, the text follows the lead of other Canadian social scientists (Coburn et al. 1987) in pushing for new ways of talking and thinking about health, disease and medicine. Many, including myself, think that Canada is at a crossroads in health care. We may choose the road back to private medical care, following the lead of Britain, or the road to "business medicine" as in the United States. In the interets of better health for all Canadians, we must see criticism of the current state of health care as a positive step. This book is neither a personal attack on physicians nor a call for the abolition of the present system. It is simply an appeal for more social awareness of an issue critical to all Canadians.

Notes

1. For the sake of grammatical simplicity, I use "he" to refer to doctors and "she" to refer to patients, although of course there are many female doctors and many male patients.

Acknowledgments

This sociology of medicine text was developed from my lectures at the University of Winnipeg. I am grateful to all my students at the university, especially the honours students in my medical sociology class, and to those nursing students at the Health Sciences Centre and Grace Hospital who were in my sociology classes. Their contributions and questions assisted greatly in the writing of this text. Particularly, I would like to thank Patricia Birk, Ray Foui and Les Tichroew. I am grateful to Vivienne Walters for helping to organize my thoughts on medical sociology and to Janet Turner who convinced me that I could write this text. Michael Wahn listened to my questions and spent valuable time with me discussing the form and content of the text. Kathleen Hamilton is to be thanked for putting my prose into a readable form. The University of Winnipeg supplied me with financial support and the Department of Sociology provided encouragement. The staff at Butterworths were very supportive and made this task relatively pleasant. Lastly, I would like to thank Fiona Green and Max for their emotional support.

Table of Contents

List of Boxes

List of Figures

List of Tables

Chapter 1

Sociology and Medicine

Introduction

Health is becoming one of the greatest concerns of Canadians. Many of us live with the fear of becoming ill and the hope that medical science will calm this fear. We are constantly being made aware of potentially life-enhancing discoveries in medicine, such as artificial hearts, while being frightened by the outbreak of new diseases, for example AIDS, and the potential harm from industrial and environmental threats. Our health and our perceptions of health are being transformed by what is happening in the society around us. What happens to the Canadian population in general touches each one of us individually.

As sociologists have shown, our lives are connected within sets of social relationships through our work, personal and family life, and day-to-day activities. Any disruption of these relationships, such as that caused by unemployment, can adversely affect our health (D'Arcy and Siddique 1985). We also know that our state of health affects our ability to participate in our social networks. There is a growing concern in Canada not only about health and illness, but about the quality of life.[1]

We are constantly being reminded by sources ranging from the federal government to television advertisements that we should take responsibility for our own health by committing ourselves to a healthy lifestyle, or to wellness (Ardell 1985). Responsibility for health as well as medication (**over-the-counter drugs**) and personal testing (e.g. for pregnancy) is being shifted from the medical and social spheres onto the individual. Health care costs, too, are being shifted from the public sector to the individual and family.

This shift toward emphasis on individual responsibility for health care is having a dramatic effect on our perceptions of, and demands for, traditional medical care, while giving us less control over the potential social causes of ill health. The faulty assumption that individuals control their lives, independently of their social context, leads to blaming the victims for their misfortunes. For example, cancer prevention efforts focus on the individual's **lifestyle**, instead of looking at environmental pollution as a cause of cancer. Status relationships between receivers and givers of health care are being reinforced (Fisher and Todd 1986, xiii).

Our culture and history have influenced the general perception of health as an individual responsibility. It seems natural, then, that we should each be responsible for our own health, as we are for our other actions. However, this book takes the perspective that we must look to social, as well as individual, prevention.

Pressure to increase individual responsibility for health is resulting not only from the inability of medicine to cure the diseases of modern civilization, cancer and heart disease, but also from society's inability to pay for the proposed cures. There is a shrinking of the resources and funds available to meet the growing demand for medical services. As a consequence, we are now moving into an era of diminished medical responsibility and, paradoxically, an increased reliance on medical expertise. The situation is further aggravated by the recent push by physicians to gain control over the supply of health care and demand whatever people are willing to pay for it.

The focus on individual responsibility sees the person, or patient, as a consumer in a supermarket of medical choices. The patient "shops" for suppliers to fill her medical needs. (For the sake of grammatical simplicity I will use "she" to refer to patients and "he" to refer to doctors, although of course there are many female doctors and many male patients.) Many supporters of this model see health as a commodity and assert that if we had less government control of medicine we would have better medicine (Blomquist 1979). Their assumption is that the consumer, by choosing "good" medicine, would eventually force bad medicine or quackery out of business. This model also assumes that individuals have to take care of themselves and be held responsible for the causes and costs of their sickness or disability. However, in a world of unregulated competition, only the wealthy could afford the benefits of medical knowledge. It is a fact that the wealthy in Canada live longer and are healthier than the poor, and this gap would grow larger in the marketplace model described above.[2]

However, health is not a commodity to be bought and sold, and patients are not consumers of health care in the same way shoppers are consumers of goods. The health care system should not be used as an instrument to separate the rich from the poor; wealth should not equal health. Health should not be the monopoly of a single group in society, the medical profession. Health care is part of the public sphere and should be administered by the representatives of the population, that is, the State, for the good of the whole population.

In the past ten years a new discourse about health has developed

(Fisher and Todd 1986; Mishler 1984)[3], which in part reflects a movement popular at the turn of the 20th century, called Social Medicine (Sand 1952). This discourse still uses the language and perspective of traditional medical practice, but centres on the lifestyle or wellness of the individual, rather than the society's effect on individual health. Ill health is seen as something we could remedy if we chose to, not something having social origins and therefore social solutions. This medical discourse, which supports the market model and the concept of individual responsibility, can be found in the reports, journals, books, government reports and other documents which deal with the health of the population. It offers methods and criteria to define cause, treatment, and cure, thus invalidating the layperson's right to enter this area.

This medical discourse allows physicians to exert control and power over their patients through the definition of health and the treatment of symptoms. "Doctors' power, consistent with our current medical model, is organized to control medical resources and influence patients' health" (Fisher and Todd 1986, x). This professional power manifests itself in two kinds of process, which are interdependent. There is the macro-process, in which physicians are supported by institutional structures (government, professional organizations, hospitals and clinics), and the micro-process, where the doctor's power is maintained and expressed in interpersonal interactions and patient control. "The power the medical profession has over the population of patients is a political reality realized and reflected in social actions which in turn often help to support the status quo" (Fisher and Todd 1986, xiii).

It may seem that Canada enjoys the health benefits of a good standard of living and a good medical care system. Many university students, who are a privileged group in Canada, see that health care is easily available in this country, that the standards are high and that everyone is treated equally by the health care system. However, these perceptions are superficial and need closer examination. Such an examination cannot be based solely on our personal experiences, good or bad, but must extend to include all groups in the population. Only by treating the study of health and health care critically can we help to advance the health of the Canadian population.

The purpose of this text is to provide the background from which questions can be asked about how this discourse and the present organizational and institutional structures influence the health of Canadians. The basic assumption is that health is *necessary* for our lives and therefore should be guaranteed to all. Our goal, as Canadians, should be to ensure the best possible standard of health for everyone in our society. Therefore, we must think of possible alternatives to the present health-care system.

Issues of Concern

In any historical period, popular notions of health and illness are influenced by contemporary medical thinking (King 1982). Non-medical approaches to health care are neither supported by the medical profession nor sanctioned by the State. For example, midwifery is a traditional form of medical care used extensively in many countries, but it has been discouraged by the medical establishment in Canada until recently, and is only now starting a comeback, under medical control (Cann et al. 1987). To break this pattern of control by the medical establishment, we must start from the beginning and look at health and medicine in a new way which will expand our vision of health, disease and illness in Canada.

First of all, we must realize that our society's present method of curing and healing, called **allopathic** medicine, is but one method of treating illness and disease, and not the only method. (*Allopathy* is a system of medical practice that treats diseases "by methods of drugs antagonistic to the manifestations of the disease being treated" (Walton et al. 1986 Vol. 1, 39). Allopathy is used to describe orthodox medicine today. One alternative to allopathic medicine is *homeopathic* medicine, which emphasizes the relationship between the parts and whole of the person. Popular and folk medicine also play a role in the treatment of illness. Zola (1972) estimated that 70% to 90% of recognized symptoms of illness are managed by individuals outside the present formal system of health care.) Although allopathic medicine has been and will continue to be of great benefit to individuals and society, this form of medical practice can also be harmful (Illich 1976). In fact, the greatest health benefits to a society are more environmental than medical: ". . . the real reasons for the vast improvement in the health of the western world have had more to do with improved living conditions, than our modern curative medical system" (Vavasour and Mennie ND, Section 1). Many diseases prevalent in the nineteenth century were eliminated *prior* to the advent of scientific medical practice, simply by better housing, food, water and working conditions (McKeown 1979).

In the case of tuberculosis, medical science and practice did have a resounding effect in lowering the rates of mortality (McKeown 1979, 96-97). However, it cannot be ignored that medical intervention was preceded by the reduction of malnutrition and overcrowding, which had made tuberculosis so formidable in the 19th century.

McKeown (1979, 197) shows that the intervention of medicine in the disease process has accounted for much less of a drop in mortality rates and increase in life expectancy than we would think: "The improvement of health in the last three centuries was due essentially to provision of food, protection from hazards, and limitation of numbers [population]". He goes on to say ". . . the therapeutic advances of the last few decades have had little effect on death rates, and that in developed countries we are approaching the 'normal' lifespan which medicine cannot be expected to extend" (1979, 191).

FIGURE 1.1

RESPIRATORY TUBERCULOSIS: MEAN ANNUAL DEATH-RATES (STANDARDIZED TO 1901 POPULATION): ENGLAND AND WALES

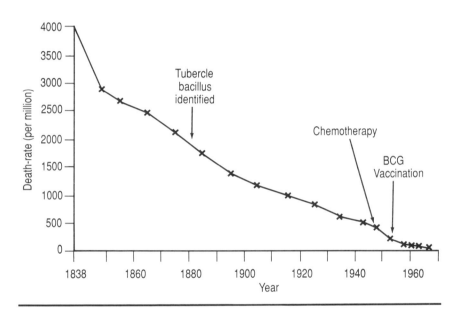

SOURCE: Thomas McKeown, *The Role of Medicine: Dream, Mirage or Nemesis?* Copyright ©
1979 Princeton University Press. Fig. 8.1 reprinted with permission of
Princeton University Press.

Oddly enough, while it is generally accepted that improvements in the environment and living conditions have in the past benefited people's health, it is considered controversial today to mention these factors when talking of the current health differences between different social classes and ethnic groups. Today, the primary focus of medical research is on the particular genetic or hereditary characteristics of individuals, rather than on the social ecology of a particular group.

The dominance of the medical model in the treatment of illness in Canada does not mean that everyone holds or agrees with this model, even within the medical profession. If the medical profession and its view of health and illness are dominant, it is because, as an institutionalized system, it organizes, shapes, guides and influences the practice of medicine and the definition of health. This dominance is also legitimized through legislation, since the medical profession is granted a monopoly by the government.

Our acceptance of and demand for medical services only reinforce medical dominance over the definition of health and over those who need medical assistance. According to Fisher and Todd (1986), the structural strength of the medical institution is intertwined with its professional control over knowledge and medical language, a control that leaves the patient dependent on the physician and the type of medicine the physician practises.

In our analysis of health we do not want to abandon medical knowledge and treatment, but to limit it to its area of expertise. We want to expand the concept of health to consider social relations as part of illness and its treatment. (In theory this is what should always happen but many patients, fearful and in ill health, are influenced by the power of the physician. They may be intimidated by threats like "It's your responsibility then" if they are reluctant to take the physician's advice.)

This book takes the position that our health is not something that can be narrowly defined, but is a complex formed by the relation between larger issues of health and illness, the medical system, the environment, and our personal experience of illness.

This experience does not always correspond with the medical definition of the illness (Kleinman et al. 1978, 251). The experience of pain, for example, goes beyond the scientific definitions of disease and biochemical treatments. Our personal experience of illness will depend on our social position, class, gender, ethnicity and cultural history. Health and illness, we will see, are social and not individual problems:

> disease and its treatment are only in the abstract purely biological processes . . . such facts as whether a person gets sick at all, what kinds of disease he acquires and what kind of treatment he receives depend largely on social factors. (Ackerknecht in Lieban 1977, 14)

The goal of this text is neither to reach a universal, unchanging definition of health and illness, nor to provide all possible interpretations of the information. Rather, the goal is (1) to allow for the questioning of current definitions of health, disease and medicine, and (2) to develop a more holistic approach which ". . . illustrates the influence of human relations on human activities, abilities, and attributes in a way which challenges established 'common sense' prejudice and which does not reject, but makes use of, biological and psychological knowledge" (Hirst and Woolley 1982, viii).

The following section will introduce the field of medical sociology.

The discussion will then proceed to definitions of health, illness and disease, taking into consideration the conflicts between medical/biological definitions and social/cultural definitions.[4]

Sociology and Medicine

Sociology and medicine[5] are distinct disciplines with distinct histories and traditions, although both are relatively young. Each has its own set of goals, concepts, jargon, and logic. The concern of medicine is the elimination of disease in society and the betterment of the health of individuals. For the most part, the focus of medicine, or object of analysis, is the individual, rather than society. This focus determines the definition and treatment of problems within the doctor/patient relationship. Sociology, on the other hand, has broader concerns (Zeitlin 1984). Even though there is a social problems[6] orientation to some sociological research, the main concern of sociology is to gain an understanding of social interaction. As we know, sociology's object of study is social relationships, or the relations between individuals within a particular social structure. (These are referred to as *lived social relations*.) The sociology of medicine applies this focus to the study of the medical establishment as part of society.

The following comparison between sociology and medicine will focus on the methods of each and how each studies problems and arrives at conclusions and recommendations for better health and health care. Since both medicine and sociology are concerned about the relation between health and illness, we can begin by looking at the natural history of a disease as outlined by Mausner and Kramer (1985, 7-9).

The Natural History of a Disease

"Disease is seen as a neutral and natural entity residing in nature, that is, in the body of the patient" (Turner 1987, 2). Any disease goes through a process of growth and decline. The stages in this process are longer for **chronic** diseases and shorter for **acute** diseases. The point at which a person is considered to have a disease depends on a number of factors; there is no absolute definition which applies to every case. The history of a disease is important for medicine since it defines the stages at which medicine can intervene to prevent or control it. There are four stages in the history of any disease: (1) susceptibility; (2) presymptomatic stage; (3) clinical disease; and (4) disability or recovery. The ideal for clinical practice is to intervene as early as possible in the history of a disease; however, in practice this is not the case.

The first stage, susceptibility, applies to the entire population at risk. For example, people who smoke are at risk of getting (are susceptible to) lung cancer, but not everyone who smokes will get lung cancer. The second, or presymptomatic stage is when the disease begins to manifest itself but still goes undetected by the medical profession and the patient. Ideally the medical practitioner would like to start intervention at this stage, to catch the disease before it gains strength; however, this is difficult when there is no evidence that the disease is present. The third stage, clinical disease, is when the disease is manifest in the individual and the doctor attempts to control the development of the disease, or cure it. This is the point at which the patient enters the statistical profile of the specific disease. The last stage, disability or recovery, occurs when the disease has run its course and the sufferer is either cured or disabled. Disability means that the individual can no longer continue functioning normally at work or in familial and personal relationships.

FIGURE 1.2

SCHEMATIC REPRESENTATION OF THE NATURAL HISTORY OF A DISEASE

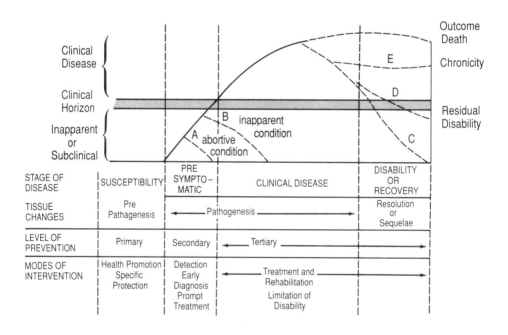

SOURCE: J.S. Mausner and S. Kramer, *Epidemiology: An Introductory Text.* Toronto: W.B. Saunders, 1985. P. 6-13.

The Clinical Method

Allopathic medicine has two main branches, research (the theoretical) and clinical practice (the practical, or applied). The clinical method is based on the concept that an individual's disease is defined by a single symptom or a complex of signs or symptoms. These signs point to an entity which must be controlled or eliminated through medical intervention, before the individual can be restored to health. This concept is sometimes referred to as the "germ theory" of disease. (The germ theory can be criticized for failing to see the body as a complex system of interactive parts which can be influenced by the social-psychological state of the individual. Alternative types of medicine are discussed in Chapter 7. Holism is defined in Chapter 2.)

Once a new disease is defined, the biological sciences[7] take up the task of locating the **cause**, or studying the **etiology**, of the disease. The disease is finally labelled and listed in the *International Classification of Diseases* (ICD), put out by the World Health Organization, according to the symptoms which are the signs of that disease.[8] Clinical medicine, as an applied science, rather than a theoretical science, builds upon the experience of cases and is in a state of constant change and reformulation; therefore, the ICD is periodically revised and updated.

Medical anthropologists point out that modern methods of disease classification tend to use one **taxonomic** system[9] for all diseases. This system of classification is used as a *transcultural* reference for the diagnosis of disease (Lieban 1977, 22) – in other words, it assumes that there is little cultural, historical or social variation in the definition of disease.[10] Cultural or social factors are not seen as important since scientists think diseases are universal, biological phenomena that are not influenced by social and cultural variation.

Clinical examination or diagnosis is concerned with linking the symptoms or signs to a disease. Totman (1979, 27), however, points out that the search for a single cause is misleading:

> Suppose an individual says that he feels alternatively hot and cold, and that his muscles ache and his throat is sore. His doctor diagnoses 'flu. Implicit in this diagnosis is the belief that the patient is infected with a 'flu virus which has caused his immune system to react in a particular predictable manner, giving rise, in turn, to the symptoms which he feels. A chain of causes and effects, having several discrete stages, from entry of the virus to the experience and report of the symptoms, is assumed to have taken place.

Figure 1.3 shows the model on which this assumption is based.

FIGURE 1.3

CAUSE/EFFECT RELATIONSHIP IN DISEASE

invasion of virus $\longrightarrow$ response of $\longrightarrow$ symptoms (sore
                            immune system   throat, aches, etc.)

SOURCE: R. Totman, *The Social Causes of Illness.* London: Souvenir Press, 1979. P. 27.

Totman goes on to say that this model is simplistic because there may be a number of reasons why a person has the 'flu. He suggests a more complex model, shown in Figure 1.4, that includes factors *preceding* the invasion of the virus in Figure 1.3 (1979, 28):

FIGURE 1.4

EXTENDED CAUSE/EFFECT RELATIONSHIP IN DISEASE

a)   genetic susceptibility
b)   concentration of antigens impinging
                                 $\longrightarrow$ Figure 1.3
c)   repertoire of antibodies
d)   status of the immune system

SOURCE: R. Totman, *The Social Causes of Illness.* London: Souvenir Press, 1979. P. 28.

With reference to this more complex model, the intention of medical practice is to intervene in the chain of events between cause and manifestation of the symptom, since the development of the virus cannot be reversed. Therefore, medical practice is not as clear-cut as it would seem.

It should be borne in mind that clinical practice, unlike medical research, is not always carried out on the basis of scientific principles. In many ways, clinical practice involves the "art" of medicine, or the ability to soothe the patient and facilitate health.

We can see this "art" in the prescription of broad-spectrum drugs to cover the many possible types of 'flu the patient may have.[11] Many times physicians define a disease (make a diagnosis) according to the **drug** that cures it. When the diagnosis is uncertain, a drug is prescribed to cover a number of possibilities, and if the drug works the possibilities are narrowed down. One drug after another may be tried. This means that patients are being used to test a specific treatment, so that each becomes a case study. In the quest to find the cause of the disease, through analysis of the symptoms, curing the patient becomes secondary. The clinical intervention may even cause pain and suffering to the patient by testing and research. Since there is no cure for some diseases, such as advanced cancers, many forms of surgery and medical treatment are experimental. The rationale for such treatments is then to enhance or perfect medical knowledge, not to cure the patient. Many times no treatment at all is as good as surgery (Bulkely and Ross 1978).

A clinical consultation, following the above model, goes as follows. The search for a disease is started when the patient presents herself to the physician with a specific complaint. This complaint is usually viewed as a symptom of some condition. It is the job of the physician to distinguish among all the possible causes of the patient's symptoms. Second, the physician seeks more information by asking the patient about the symptom and possibly about the patient's life, to find out whether there may be some work- or home-related cause of the problem. For example, working with asbestos or being unemployed could both cause illness. (It is not known whether lifestyle information actually has any effect on the treatment prescribed. Physicians are under constraints as to how much they can do for their patients. They usually don't prescribe a change of job or residence, if these are not viable alternatives.) After a general diagnosis is made, the physician may order tests (e.g. blood and urine tests) to confirm the diagnosis. Third, the physician prescribes a treatment, which may be in keeping with the accepted view of how the symptoms should be dealt with, or else tailored to suit the type of patient or personal view of the physician. The former is usually the case. Finally, the **prognosis** is made. This is the future or result the patient has to look forward to, an indication as to whether and when the symptoms will be relieved. The prognosis is based on general averages of the past success of the treatment on other patients with similar symptoms. Throughout this process, the patient plays a passive role and is little more than the host of the disease.

Diagnosis is probably the most interpretive part of medical practice, and the reason why many physicians call medicine an "art." With the development of more and more diagnostic technology, physicians are relying on tests and computerized diagnosis instead of their own experiences.[12] However, some studies show that the use of technology in diagnosis is inversely related to correct diagnosis: ". . . the percentage of correct diagnosis actually is declining in many hospitals, despite the development of CAT scanners, ultrasound, and other sophisticated diagnostic equipment" (American Funeral Director 1984). Reliance on technology and testing does little to develop the individual human abilities of the physician, which in turn results in a need for more technology.

Since the beginning of the 19th century, the medical search for the cause of disease has shifted from the social nature of symptoms, to the individual's tissues, and finally to the chemistry of cells and tissues. It could be said, in fact, that the focus of medicine has shifted from the individual to the component parts of the individual (Starr 1982).[13]

There is always a risk within clinical practice that a dangerous method or drug will be used. A number of deaths may occur before the use of the drug is discontinued. One problem is that the effects may be long-term, and the fatal consequences discovered only years after, when it is too late to help those who have taken the drug. An example of this is diethylstilbestrol (DES), which produced cancer in the *daughters* of the women who had taken it. Another example is thalidomide, which was given to pregnant women to prevent nausea, and which caused their children to be born without limbs.

In theory, every drug and medical technique should be tested before being used on humans. In fact, even after testing, there are always risks associated with medical treatment. Even where the risks of a given treatment may be small, there are patients who will die from that treatment.

In other words, patients are used to test whether or not certain practices or drugs are harmful. Many of the various drugs and techniques used to control or alter reproduction have proved fatal to women who accepted their doctor's advice (Stanworth 1987).

Since 1967 brain bypass surgery has been used on stroke patients, who number 5,000 annually in North America, to restore blood flow to the impaired section of the brain and thus facilitate functioning. Recent information suggests however that this operation is useless and in many cases actually increases the patient's risk of stroke.[14]

Some may argue that these deaths and defects are necessary or justified because of the benefits offered by the successful techniques (Banagale 1984). But are there really gains in the long run? And should we, as patients, all be subjects of clinical experiments? There are moral and ethical issues here as well as biological issues. Should the medical profession have the right to try and extend the life of a person, if the process may be harmful? Is living better than dying if it means being confined to a bed and made dependent on drugs and technology? Physicians have little training in these moral and ethical issues.

In looking at the clinical method we must remember that the elimination of symptoms does not necessarily mean the termination of disease. It has been argued that a great deal of medical practice is concerned with the elimination of pain rather than disease, and that physicians are treating the product and not the cause of the ailment.

In light of the above, we should begin to ask ourselves how much of the clinical model of health and illness is incorporated into our own perceptions or self-analysis of our signs or symptoms? Do we treat these symptoms in a way that is similar to medical practice? What do we see as the sources or cause of these symptoms?

The Sociological Method

As stated above, the central assumption of the clinical method is that symptoms are caused either by a malfunction in the body or by a disease. It could be said that the problem with the medical approach is its (narrow) scope, or the factors it takes into account. Even though medical students are taught to uncover all possible reasons for illness, they overlook many of the social and psychological reasons for illness since they are not within the scope of the medical model or "hard" science. To contrast, a sociological approach would not rule out symptoms, but would attempt to expand the scope of the search for cause.

> In medicine, when the cause of a disease is identified it represents a choice from a wide selection of possible causal factors, both in type and over time. The contribution of the behavioural sciences to an understanding of disease aetiology [cause] is to claim neither that the new explanations of behavioural science are better nor that the more common biological explanations are wrong. (Armstrong 1980, 54)

In contrast to the clinical method, which focuses narrowly on the individual, the sociological method treats health and illness as "social facts" that have social definitions and define constraints on our behaviour (Giddens 1971, 86-89). Sociologists do not ignore the fact that it is the individual who experiences the illness, but they are more concerned with the relations within which the illness is experienced. Sociologists seek answers to questions about the **prevalence** and **incidence**[15] of specific diseases in a particular **population**. They attempt to find out how social factors may relate to how long we live, what diseases we will contract and how we will be treated when we are ill.

Do specific ethnic groups have a high incidence of a particular disease? Are individuals working in a particular job showing similar patterns of symptoms? Do hospitals and medical practitioners cause illness and suffering? To answer these questions we must look beyond individuals to their social relationships (Rose et al. 1985b, Introduction). Sociology, then, studies the patterns of individual and group relations. In order to explain social behaviour and forms of social organization, such as that of hospitals and professions, generalizations are made by interpreting the interactions of individuals within or between these spheres.

Sociology as a discipline tries to understand the dynamics of change and transformation (Giddens 1982). There are various possible sociological perspectives, which flow from the theoretical models of the "fathers" of sociology, Marx, Weber and Durkheim. This book takes a generally critical (rather than functional or mainstream) perspective which allows for progress and change in the present way we think of health and practise health care. (This text is written for students who have had an introductory sociology course. For an outline of the different sociological theories as they apply to medicine, see Bond and Bond 1986, Chapter 2.)

The general assumption of sociology is that individuals cannot be understood outside their social relationships since individuals are shaped by the interactions of which they are a part. The focus of sociological research is the relation between the individual and his or her environment or network. Since individuals are embedded in a network of relations which not only influence their health but also their conceptions of health and illness, we must focus on these relations in studying health and illness. Although the tendency of sociology since Durkheim has been to view the individual as a product of social factors (Hirst and Woolley 1982, viii), this text does not see the individual as being manipulated by the larger "social system" or having little control over his or her life. In fact, the social environment which surrounds the individual can also be shaped by the individuals within it. We live within a set of constraints but those constraints are not immutable. Individuals, then, have a personal politics within a given set of social constraints (Henriques et al. 1984). That is, they are able, to a greater or lesser extent, to influence their social situation.

Social scientists look at the impact that a disease or biological "cause" has on individuals within a network of relationships, and also at the social situation which may foster or check the disease (Williams 1980, 84).

Individuals cope with illness in different ways, depending on their social environment and relationships. The length and severity of a disease influence social relationships and, in turn, these relationships can influence the length and severity of a disease.

> Physical or mental impairments can affect people in a very large number of ways: disease can limit or modify the range of normal activities, as can its treatment; acute attacks of illness may remove an individual from ordinary life entirely; . . . disease renders people abnormally conscious of their physical or mental condition; many sufferers are stigmatised by others; disease may be a regular source of pain or anxiety, which may in turn affect relations with others. (Rose et al. 1985b, 61)

If an individual is stigmatized (Goffman 1963) by having a certain disease, such as epilepsy, this stigmatization affects the person's ability to cope with the disease and live a normal life. The stress and anxiety of a particular situation can in turn make people more susceptible to certain diseases (Dilley et al. 1985). Being a member of a socially stigmatized group, such as homosexuals, can put an individual more at risk of getting certain diseases. Of course it is difficult to prove which comes first, the biological or the social situation. In fact, the separation of the biological and the social spheres may be the wrong way to approach the study of illness and disease. Before going any further, it is important to look at the difference between *disease* and *illness*.

Disease and Illness: Definitions

The medical view of disease and illness is summed up by Dr. Anthony Reading (1977, 703) as follows:

> The terms *illness* and *disease* lack precision. . . . Illness tends to be used to refer to what is wrong with the patient, disease is what is wrong with his body. *Illness* is what the patient suffers from, what troubles him, what he complains of, and what prompts him to seek medical attention. Illness refers to the patient's *experience* of ill-health. It comprises his impaired sense of well being, his perception that something is wrong with his body, and his various symptoms of pain, distress, and disablement. *Disease*, on the other hand, refers to various structural disorders of the individual's tissues and organs that give rise to the signs of ill-health. These are, for the most part, not accessible to the patient and not experienced by him. Disease may thus exist for considerable periods of time without the patient knowing. (Reading 1977, 703)

From a sociological point of view, a *disease* is defined as a structural disorder of an individual's tissues and organs that gives rise to symptoms of ill health. *Illness* is the state of being unable to function in society because of health reasons. Illness refers to the individual's social world, while *disease* refers to the person's physiological system (Spradlin and Porterfield 1979, 139). We can have a disease without acting ill, and we can act as if we are ill without having a disease.

> Similar degrees of organ pathology may generate quite different reports of pain and distress; illness may occur in the absence of disease (50% of visits to the doctor are for complaints without an ascertainable biologic base); and the course of the disease is distinct from the trajectory of the accompanying illness. (Kleinman et al. 1978, 251-52)

Although illness is a social behaviour and disease is a biological phenomenon, either may affect the other. When we are ill we have to act accordingly, so those around us can acknowledge that we are ill and treat us appropriately. Since the physician, using the clinical method, relies on symptoms or signs to know that a person is ill, then these signs must be manifest in individuals. These symptoms must also be communicated to and accepted by the doctor.

> . . . changes in the study of illness behaviour have been marked by a shift away from an emphasis on explaining behaviour in terms of medical rationality, towards attempting to understand the lay person's actions in terms of their own logic, knowledge and beliefs. . . . This change in image of the lay person appears to pose considerable practical problems for the medical profession. For example, it has been argued (Armstrong 1984) that the discovery that lay theories about disease are both rational and theoretically sophisticated necessitates a change in clinical practice in at least two ways. The first involves a change in technique in that good clinical practice should involve considering and responding to the patients' theories about illness, and not just being concerned with diagnosis and treatment. . . . The second requires a more fundamental change, in that it involves a reassessment of the value of the conceptual framework used in present-day clinical practice. (Morgan et al. 1985, 103-4)

Medical practitioners have problems with the mix of social and biological factors in the many variations of illness behaviour. "A doctor . . . need not be aware of the social basis of disease to practice medicine though this does not mean that medicine is other than a social enterprise" (Armstrong 1983, 73). Confusion in diagnosis, for the physician, is brought about by a reliance on the "Doctrine of Specific Aetiology: a specific disease always has a specific cause" (Hart 1985, 14).

Types of Disease

There are two general categories of disease: **communicable** and non-communicable. Communicable diseases are a threat to the health of individuals and the entire population. They may be caused by a variety of organisms. The problem for medicine is their identification and treatment. The search is for the agent of the disease, a source, and the way it is transmitted. Usually the life span of communicable diseases is short, and they are repelled by the body's immune system. Some examples of communicable diseases are measles, mumps and AIDS. Non-communicable diseases are not transferred from person to person, but are our major causes of death. Examples include cancer and heart disease.

Both communicable and non-communicable diseases can be either acute or chronic. Acute disease is marked by a sharp or severe change in the individual's health. It has a rapid onset and comes rapidly to a conclusion. Clinical medicine has had much success with acute disease, and indeed specializes in it; the clinical model is based upon acute disease. Chronic disease is long-term and may be an unknown disease, multiple diseases or natural degeneration of the body through old age. Medical attention is usually inadequate in the case of chronic disease and the treatment is custodial. The chronically ill pose a problem for medicine since their numbers are increasing as the population ages and they occupy a large proportion of hospital beds. Chronic disease also has a substantial effect on the sufferers, their self-perceptions and their relationships with their family.

As stated above, the focus of medicine is to find the cause of the disease within the individual and then treat that disease. Sociology, however, looks more to prevention. It looks at the development and transportation of the disease, that is, at its social context, and then seeks to eliminate those social connections or situations which give rise to the disease (see Horn 1969 and Zinsser 1935).

Accidents, especially motor vehicle accidents, are one of the major causes of mortality in Canada.[16] If we want to reduce the **rates** of **mortality** caused by such accidents, what measures can we take? Many would focus on drivers and require them to use seatbelts or to subject themselves to tests for alcohol and drug use. These measures may reduce the rate of accidents, but they do not eliminate them. They are only secondary methods of preventing injury. Instead we could approach the problem in larger social terms, by focusing on the relation between the use of cars as a mode of transportation and the society that views the car, for lack of alternatives, as necessary. Within this approach we would question the safety and design of the cars we drive, the roads we use, the training of drivers, and the lack of comprehensive public transport. This would be primary prevention.

Illness and the Sick Role

The definition of diseases tends to be universal, however, illness behaviour is not. For example, cancer patients from different cultures may not exhibit the same symptoms, behave in the same way or have a similar response to treatment. Sick individuals have to act as if they are sick, in a way that is socially defined as "appropriate," to get sympathy and attention from others. Individuals sometimes "play sick" for their own advantage. The sick role is a way of getting out of certain obligations: work, family responsibilities or university exams.

The bulk of sociological research on illness revolves around the sick role, or illness behaviour (Conrad and Kern 1986, 123). The concept of the sick role was developed by Parsons (1951) and has been incorporated in almost every medical sociology text. Ehrenreich and Ehrenreich (1978) and Segall (1976) have analyzed this concept at length. The following quotation will serve to define it in the light of social research.

> The characteristics of the sick role are: 1) The individual is not held responsible for his/her condition. (Sinners and criminals are responsible; sick people are not.) 2) Conditions defined as illness are seen as a legitimate basis for certain *exemptions* from normal responsibilities – "sick" people can stay home from work, be waited on, etc., depending on the severity of the incapacity. 3) The exemptions held out to sick persons are only *conditionally* legitimate, the prime condition being that the sick person recognize that sickness is an undesirable state and that he/she has an obligation to get well. 4) In our society, this is an obligation to seek competent help and to cooperate completely with the efforts of competent helpers in becoming well. (Ehrenreich and Ehrenreich 1978, 43) Copyright © 1978 by John Ehrenreich. Reprinted by permission of Monthly Review Foundation.

The sick role isolates and neutralizes people so they can escape the pressures and demands of "normal" life. Regardless of the therapeutic value of medical practice, the sick role fulfills a need to control behaviour; it functions in the interests of the social whole (society) (Trowler 1984, 175). For the sick role to work, there must be co-operation between doctor and patient, and the latter must believe that the definition of her behaviour as sick is in her best interests. But what if it is not in her best interests? Many individuals who are categorized as sick (the handicapped, for example) would rather be thought of as healthy. To define individuals as healthy means to place them within the boundaries which define normal behaviour. For example, if the blind were treated as normal, then society would be organized in a way which would not allow lack of vision to be a disability; the blind would not need special treatment since their need would be considered normal. (Imagine a society in which the majority of the people were blind!)

The Social Definitions of Health

One problem for those studying health, disease and medicine is to come up with a definition of health. You might think this strange, but try it for yourself. Before going on to the next paragraph take out a piece of paper and write down a definition of health. How do we know when a person is healthy?

The **model** you use will probably be an attempt at a scientific definition rooted in biology. Your definition might differ from those of others, depending on your background. Clearly, the definition of health is affected by our point of view, whether medical, social or other. Once you have a definition, try applying it to a classmate and see if he or she is healthy or ill. This brings us to the question: what is the basis for the different perceptions of health and illness?

We can start from the obvious statement that health is the absence of disease, or a state of well-being. The state of health, then, means simply having no disease, or "feeling okay." However, there are degrees of feeling healthy. For example, when we have a cold, we can still feel healthy enough to participate in our daily activities. Various cancers, too, can exist for long periods of time within individuals who feel healthy. Conversely, individuals can feel extremely ill without any known medical reason (this is routinely called psychosomatic illness). There seems to be no direct relation between feeling and being ill.

International organizations that study the health of the world have the same problem trying to define health (Hansluwka 1985). In 1946, the World Health Organization (WHO) defined health as ". . . a state of complete physical, mental and social well being, and not merely the absence of disease" (in Kelman 1975, 635). This definition is so far-reaching that it encompasses every facet of our lives: economic, political and social.[17] Very few people, and very few populations, are healthy according to this definition.

Social norms influence our definition of health, and the acceptable level of health will be different for different groups in the society. Many researchers have found variations in the definition of health between different social classes and ethnic groups (Apple 1960).

In the sociological sense, the definition of health may depend on your ability to perform the tasks of day-to-day life. If you can do your school work or job, or carry out your family responsibilities, then you are healthy, from a sociological point of view. If you are not able to, or need assistance, you are ill.

Of course, our ability to function in the society as healthy individuals is defined by the particular society we live in. The ability necessary to perform specific tasks, keep up social relationships and support oneself is different from society to society (Berliner 1977, 117). We can have a disease and still be able to function, although maybe not to our full capacity. In fact there is no state of absolute health.

> In any discussion of what constitutes good health the concept of disease has an important part to play. Yet whereas definitions of health involve judgments on the part of both doctor and patient which overtly involve social criteria, e.g. a sense of wellbeing, a knowledge of the nature and characteristics of disease is particular to the medical profession and is usually couched in biological terms. Patients claim to be ill, doctors decide whether they have a disease or not. Yet although doctors rarely have any problem in describing the characteristics of a specific disease there does seem to be some difficulty in defining what "disease" actually is. . . . Although most diseases undoubtedly do have a biological basis this is not sufficient to explain the nature of the disease *per se.* (Armstrong 1983, 69-70)

If the medical definition (health is the absence of disease) were broadened to the extent of the WHO definition, would physicians have extended powers to define who should be given medical attention? For example, obesity is now seen as a medical problem. Even being "over-weight" is considered deviant, a condition to be remedied (Turner 1987, 22).

Once a behaviour is labelled as abnormal, the implication is that it should be made normal. Therefore, the more types of behaviour that are labelled as abnormal, the more powerful the physicians become, since they are the legally sanctioned administrators of scientific medicine. Many sociologists have shown that we should be cautious of definitions which reduce social conditions to diseases which can only be remedied by the scientific form of medical practice (Hirst and Woolley 1982, 23). An example is mental illness:

> Attitudes towards mental illness and therapy are necessarily shaped and influenced by the prevailing political climate. In particular, attitudes towards insanity will depend a great deal on whether the state and the medical establishment are regarded as agents of social control, regulating deviance under the ideology of psychiatric help, or whether the state is seen to be the great protector of vulnerable and isolated individuals in a social system where the traditional supports of the family and the community are in many industrial societies in a stage of rapid decline and collapse. (Turner 1987, 81)

Disabled members of our society *can* be productive in certain types of work, but they may not be capable of doing profitable work. "Disabled" can be defined as "unable to complete the task according to the way it has been organized and defined."[18] Many disabled people can do productive work, but they cannot do it fast enough to be profitable. For example individuals in wheelchairs have the *ability* to work in restaurants as waiters, but the organization of serving food cannot accommodate these individuals; the job is not structured for people without the use of their legs. Therefore they are considered not able to do the task.

Functional health (as opposed to medical health) can thus be defined as the ability to be a productive member of the society, or the type of person that fits the tasks a society demands (Kelman 1975, 634). We must realize that the social structure in which we live and the institutions in which we work affect both the definition of functional health and our capacity for participation (Dreitzel 1971, xi).

Another way of defining health is according to the degree that people can control their own destiny (Kelman 1975; Berliner 1977). For example, if we are poor and live in a situation of high stress, with a high risk of getting ill, then our ability to fulfill the demands placed on us is limited and we feel unhealthy. If our material situation (income, housing, prospects) were to improve, we would probably experience a great improvement in our health. People may be *alienated* by knowing that they have no future, and keeping healthy may therefore have little meaning for them. Also, people's health may be affected if they are denied adequate or accurate information about the causes of ill-health.[19]

The medical profession in Canada has a monopoly control over the definition of health and illness, and benefits monetarily from its monopoly. Since the medical profession has the power to define illness and treat those who are ill, it also has the power to organize our behaviour in certain ways. Specific treatments can affect the way we organize our lives and relationships.

[Treatments] . . . are justified by the ethic of professionalization, which decrees that doctors are the exclusive owners of expert knowledge. They do not need to tell anyone else what they are doing or why. Indeed, retention of absolute control over technical procedures is clearly an absolute necessity for the survival of modern medical power. . . . Doctors' control over information available to patients is part of the defence of expert professional knowledge – never a simple act of patronage or nastiness, but absolutely intrinsic to the claim of professionalization. (Oakley 1987, 46)

Historical (Torrance 1987) and cross-cultural studies (Landy 1977) show that there is no universal definition of health and illness. In fact, definitions of health are culture-bound: the ways in which healers and sick individuals speak of "illness" are revealing about the culture in question, and its ideas of "normal" or "well" behaviour. For example, a Canadian death certificate shows a list of possible "causes of death," or explanations of the end of a person's physical existence. These possible causes refer to conditions within the body, but do *not* include social causes of these conditions, such as air pollution or stress.

In summary, defining health is problematic. If we are to study health we have to *operationalize* the **concept** (that is, develop a measure for health) so we can separate the healthy from the ill. An operational definition is crucial in making decisions about the general health of the population, and recommendations for the introduction or withdrawal of various health policies and services. Whose definition of health/illness should we accept? Defining an individual or group as ill has consequences for that individual or group.

The Sociology in and of Medicine

In medical sociology there are two avenues or approaches: (1) the sociology *of* medicine and (2) sociology *in* medicine. The distinction between the two approaches lies not in the framework or methods they use to analyze health and medicine, but rather in their theoretical assumptions.

According to Strauss (1957), the sociology *of* medicine is the study of the social organization of medicine viewed from *outside* the medical system. On the other hand, sociology *in* medicine is practised by sociologists within medical schools who assist in understanding illness and disease according to various social factors. Those working in the sociology *of* medicine are solving problems dictated by the discipline of sociology, and those working in sociology *in* medicine are solving problems dictated by medicine. Note that both types have training (usually a Ph. D.) in sociology, not in medicine.[20]

Obviously, the types of questions that may be raised within each discipline are influenced by the general purpose of that discipline and its institutional support. For example, questions asked by the "of" group might be based on the assumption that the type of medical care that exists in Canada is harmful as well as beneficial, and that the community, rather than the medical profession, should have control over health decisions. Therefore, this group would conclude, what is needed to improve the population's health or access to care is a re-organization of medical practice and a rethinking of the current definitions of health and illness (Turner 1987). Conversely, research by the "in" group would be guided by the questions the medical profession considered important. It would therefore not focus on the implications of certain social relationships; changes in this area would be ignored or thought impossible. The medical profession might see as contrary to its interests any transformation in the type of care given, or in the definition of health interests. An example might be the introduction of nurse practitioners who would be able to replace doctors. In addition, larger socio-economic and political interests might prohibit the medical profession from publicizing certain findings, for example warnings about the relation between smoking and cancer (Warner 1985).

A third example is that there is no research on home births being done in Canada by sociologists working within the medical profession; the practice of home birth is viewed with scepticism and hostility by most physicians, as shown by the following excerpt from the Canadian Medical Association's policy:

> Home deliveries cannot be justified in the light of present medical knowledge. The safeguards afforded by hospital-based obstetric care greatly surpass personal dissatis-faction with hospital policies and procedures. . . . The Canadian Medical Association believes that a planned home delivery in the absence of the full range of normally available hospital facilities can jeopardize the safety of both mother and infant. (Canadian Medical Association 1982)

Those who work to promote home births, such as Susan L. Meyer, coordinator of the Ontario Home Birth Working Group, receive little support from the medical profession, or from government.[21]

It should be pointed out that the difference between the two approaches is not that one is critical and the other conservative, since a sociologist can be critical of the medical profession from within either approach. There may be some conflict between these two approaches, especially over the cause and treatment of illness. This conflict arises from the differing assumptions, goals and limits of the conceptual bases of the researchers or their institutional settings.

When illness is defined as having a biological, chemical or physiological cause, then remedies are sought within this model.

However, when illness is defined as having an origin in social relations, then social remedies must be found. One way to resolve this conflict would be to change the focus of analysis from disease to health. Enlarging the area of research and building a sociology *of* health, not defined or controlled by the medical discourse, would work for the better health of the population.[22]

While sociology *in* medicine has received more research attention in Canada than the other approach, this text follows the approach of the sociology *of* medicine, in seeing illness as a social issue.

The Problem of Cause

The discussion of the cause of illness can be broken down into three types of explanation: the biological, the personal and the social. Within each explanation, there is a unity of (1) "cause" in the explanation of illness, and (2) the mode of intervention which fits that model of cause. In this text we will view "cause" in the context of the environment in which the disease happens; that is, there are interacting factors that constitute the "cause" of a disease (Hirst and Woolley 1982, 7).

Biological Factors (The Medical Model)

Biological explanations of illness are common in medicine, however the trouble with biological explanations is that they are *reductionist*. In other words, they oversimplify complex states and processes. Reductionism in medicine assumes that explanations for illness can be reduced to the component parts of the body. Illness is seen as the breakdown of a part; if the part is fixed, the result will be health or harmonious running of the body.

The cause of a disease, according to this model, must be located in a part of the body, and this part must be restored to "normal" functioning. This model focuses on the individual, *after* the disease is manifest. To be consistent, the treatment of the biological phenomena should be biological. However, we have seen that the clinical method intervenes only after symptoms or signs of the disease have appeared, which is late in the history of a disease.

We may have a genetic or biological predisposition to a certain ailment, such as heart disease or diabetes, but this predisposition does not mean that we will inevitably get the disease. Furthermore, it is not only wrong to use a simple biological explanation for behaviour, it is potentially harmful to refer to biology to defend certain types of behaviour, such as moral attacks on homosexuals with AIDS. Gould (1977, 258) argues that biological explanations are accepted as *truth* because they are "scientific" and therefore, by their nature, do not support any social prejudice: "This usage [of biology] is quite out of the control of individual scientists [physicians] who propose deterministic theories for a host of reasons, often benevolent." "Scientific" does not necessarily mean "correct."

The clinical model assumes that a specific disease agent was the cause of an **infection**, but there are many diseases that cannot be explained by this assumption. Humans are not isolated biological entities, but organisms embedded within a social context, a context that may be a factor in human health and illness.

Social Factors (Society as the Cause)

Today, social explanations for disease are uncommon in medicine. This has not always been the case. At the turn of the 20th century, before the heyday of drug therapy, there was a movement for a more holistic approach to medical practice (Sand 1952, 508). Although there may be some recognition of particular social factors which influence health in the 1980s, this recognition is not generally integrated into medical practice. The sociological method of analyzing the cause of disease is called *holistic*, that is, it emphasizes the relationship between the parts and the whole.

Holistic explanations describe an individual's health as part of a particular social structure and sets of social relations in which the individual is embedded. The focus of this approach is located at a point prior to the onset of a disease, since the object of study is the entire population. For example, when dealing with a population which has a high incidence of a certain disease, for example native Canadians who have high rates of tuberculosis, the holistic approach would look beyond the biological characteristics of this population to their living conditions. If the cause of the disease is social, then its treatment or prevention is social, and intervention should take place before individuals get the disease, with the intention of preventing their getting it.

Although some sociologists who use this model reject the biological basis of disease entirely, the position taken in this text is not that we should ignore the biological process of a disease, but that social aspects should be given primary importance in the analysis of health.

Personal Factors (Lifestyle)

Both the biological and social models seem to say (though in different ways) that our health is determined by forces over which we have little control. Therefore, researchers might include part of our personal history or psychological predisposition in an explanation of why we are ill or healthy. Personal or lifestyle causes are temporal, since they bring to the analysis the concept of *time*. (Note that the sequencing of cause and effect is not as simple as it may seem. In the case of an unemployed man who is depressed, for example, the depression may be a result of his job loss, or of something else entirely. The cure will depend on what the cause is thought to be.) Whatever the cause of the feelings of illness, these personal factors precede the illness in time and are seen as happening prior to the development of a disease in the medical sense. The "lifestyle explanation" of illness has become very popular in Canada since the Lalonde Report (1981).[23] It places the responsibility for good health on each one of us individually. The stress is on diet, exercise and wellness, as exemplified in the government's promotion of "Participaction." This perspective appeals to our self-control (but there is a "hidden agenda": government expenditure will be reduced if everyone adopts a healthy lifestyle).

Figure 1.5 illustrates the biological, social and personal explanations for an individual's health or illness. Although this diagram seems to indicate that the social, biological and personal factors influence us equally, in fact they all are located within a social context and each interacts with the others. These contributors are all part of the same process, having different strengths at different times.

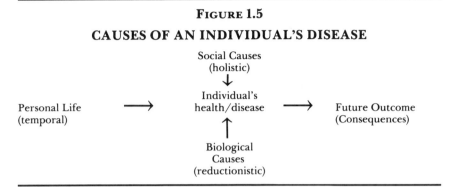

FIGURE 1.5

CAUSES OF AN INDIVIDUAL'S DISEASE

SOURCE: S. Rose et al., *Studying Health and Disease*. London: The Open University Press, 1985. P. 83.

Summary

The purpose of this chapter has been to show the difference between the medical and sociological approaches to health and illness. Definitions of health and illness have also been discussed. It should be kept in mind throughout this book that the criticism of medical practice and the medical profession has a constructive purpose: to create a better system of health care and a better social environment for health.[24] The main points of this chapter are: (1) an individual's health is influenced by his or her social environment; (2) individuals are not completely responsible for their own health; (3) the medical profession has the power to define health/illness and to decide what type of medicine will be practised and who will be able to practise it; (4) sociologists can study health and illness from inside the medical establishment or outside of its control; and (5) the sick role and the **labelling** of individuals as sick have an impact on social relationships. The succeeding chapters will develop the sociological approach by presenting a number of current issues which are changing the practice of medicine and definitions of health care in Canada.

Notes

1. "Quality of life" is a new area of research that uses complex models to define what kind of lives are good or even possible. However, it is easier to determine the quality of the environment or the quality of food than the quality of a person's life. A given individual's quality of life can be seen as good or not so good, depending on perspective.
2. Britain over the past few years has seen the introduction of a private health-care system which is drawing patients from an under-funded

National Health Service. Because of this, the gap in health between the social classes is growing (Wilkinson 1986).

3. Discourse is the language used by experts to define their field of expertise.

4. Although sociology, psychology and biology all have many good ideas and solid research to bring to the study of health and illness, the real world cannot be entirely grasped or defined according to the categories of any of these disciplines. At the present time, the biological view has gained prominence and is not only a major force in medicine but is gaining strength in the fields of psychology and sociology. Therefore this text takes a corrective approach, by pressing for the recognition of the importance of social, not only biological, processes in health and health care.

5. The term "medicine" as used in this text refers to the dominant form of medical practice in Canada, that is, scientific, allopathic medicine.

6. Within the social problems orientation the sociologist aims to solve the problems of society. Researchers in the social problems school would say that those who act to solve problems such as crime are agents of social control. These agents assist in upholding the society as it exists, for those in positions of power.

7. Biology and medicine have always been closely linked disciplines and have developed in close relation to each other, supporting each other's growth.

8. There are certain problems arising from the use of predetermined categories, such as a list of diseases. When a new disease arises, the tendency is to try to place it within the categories that are already known, and to try the treatments used for those categories. If these treatments do not work there is a search, through trial and error, for another treatment. This leads to a situation where the treatment tends to define the disease. For example, if the patient has an ailment which is not known, a positive response by the patient to a specific drug will indicate to the physician what type of disease it is. Another problem is that the use of discrete (separate) categories does not allow for the possibility of overlapping (as when there are two diseases co-existing), or masking (as when the symptoms are not related to the disease).

9. The taxonomy (i.e. classification) of diseases is done according to their biological or physiological characteristics. Medical taxonomy assumes that a patient's social characteristics (class, gender, ethnicity) have no influence on the incidence or treatment of diseases.

10. In the social sciences this is called *ethnocentrism*.

11. A common example is the prescribing of an antibiotic to a patient who has a viral infection. Many physicians say that this is done to prevent any possible problems such as development of bacterial

infections. This practice has become very controversial because the overuse of antibiotics leads to the development of resistant strains of bacteria and lowers the body's own ability to cope with bacteria.

12. There has been considerable talk of computer diagnosis; however, there is some evidence that physicians are not happy with this tool.

13. It seems as though individuals are no longer seen as whole persons but as a complex of working parts: liver, heart, brain, etc. These parts if diseased cause the person to be sick. If the parts are fixed or replaced the person will get well.

14. There is evidence that coronary bypass surgery reduces the pain of angina pectoris (chest pain) but researchers have little understanding why this is so (Bulkely and Ross 1978).

15. Prevalence is the rate of all cases of a disease, new or old, in the population. Incidence is the rate of known new cases of a disease, usually for a given year (annual rate). Both of these rates are expressed as a certain number per 100,000.

16. In the U.S.A. there have been more people killed in motor vehicle accidents than in all the wars that country has participated in since 1900.

17. Some say that if an expanded definition of health were incorporated into our health-care system, one consequence would be the expansion of the authority and power of the medical profession.

18. Even the term "disabled" is not universally defined. It has a different meaning and a different social reception according to the place and time.

19. An article by Warner (1985, 384-88) in *The New England Journal of Medicine* revealed that magazines were withholding information about the hazards of smoking in order to get large advertising contracts from the tobacco companies.

20. The sociologist *of* medicine plays a primary role in defining research, while the sociologist *in* medicine plays a secondary role. The former is like a manager, the latter like an employee.

21. It should be noted that there is a powerful medical lobby and that physicians sit on the government and other boards which give financial assistance to medical research.

22. As pointed out by Thomas Kuhn (1962), a professional group has a particular frame of reference, or paradigm, with which it views the outside world. Specific values, beliefs and perspectives are contained within this paradigm. Therefore, the paradigm sets the questions for research as well as the proposed types of answers for those questions.

23. Marc Lalonde attributed health to four factors: (1) the *human biology* element included those aspects of mental and physical health which are a direct consequence of the basic biology of the individual; (2) the *environment* element includes all those matters related to health

which are external to the human body and over which the individual has little or no personal control; (3) the *lifestyle* element includes those decisions made by individuals themselves, which have implications for their health; (4) *health care organization* consists of "the quantity, quality, arrangement, nature, and relationships of people and resources in the provision of health care" (Bond and Bond 1986, 12-13).

24. While there are many physicians within the medical profession who criticize medical orthodoxy, they are in a minority and do not control policy for the profession as a whole. Also, as individual physicians, they are constrained by their education, practice, institutional affiliations, professional membership, patients and associates. For example, there are physicians practising in Canada who have been trained in Britain and have learned homeopathy but are not allowed to practise this form of medicine in Canada.

Chapter 2

The Social Construction of Health

Today the terms "health" and "illness" are commonly understood in the medical sense. The sociological definition of health and illness is neither commonly used nor understood. To develop a sociological understanding of health we will start with the concept of social construction (Berger and Luckmann 1967). Simply put, social construction means that the society we live in determines our ideas about basic "facts" such as love, sex and death. In other words, a social interpretation is given to these issues. Our definitions of health and illness, therefore, are influenced by time and place.

> Each person considers his illness and the meaning that he assigns to it to be an individual experience and perception, which he takes to be objective and obvious. The sociologist tries to understand how this experience and perception are, in fact, a construction that transcends the individual. (Herzlich and Pierret 1985, 146)

Scientific as well as social definitions are constantly changing and reflecting the concerns of a particular culture at a specific time in history. The concept of social construction negates the notion that there are universal definitions of health and illness. Although diseases themselves are universal, the ways in which they are perceived and exhibited in behaviour are socially constructed. The biological signs of a disease can give rise to a wide variety of medical diagnoses, and there can be wide variation in the ways the illness is perceived by the sufferer (Mishler 1981).

> Our notions of health, disease, symptoms, normal functioning, illness, etc., are socially derived and an important part of the sociology of medicine is to investigate how they arose, how they are maintained and their implications for health and the health services. (Armstrong 1980, 2)

Therefore, those working within the medical system think of health and illness in ways they have been taught. Their views of health/illness are reinforced by working in a system which supports these ideas and by associating with others who think the same way.

However, differences of opinion about disease and health exist not only in the general population but also in the medical profession. Physicians from different countries may disagree on the definition of a specific ailment, especially in psychiatry. Even physicians within the same hospital will often disagree on a specific diagnosis and treatment when given the same symptoms (Koran 1975).

Medical Practice and the Social Construction of Health

As the previous chapter showed, medical science attempts to classify diseases on the basis of previous clinical experience. This approach inhibits re-ordering and ties classification to past theories of disease. According to Armstrong (1980, 70), "the disadvantage with this model is that over-adherence to a rigid classification can cause important factors which do not fall into the classification to be overlooked."

> The disease model is merely one of potentially many ways of classifying medical problems. Its advantage lies in the fact that in its long history it has been considerably refined and developed and so now provides a fairly sophisticated means of classifying problems which in turn enables treatment to be appropriately directed. (Armstrong 1980, 70)

In Box 2.1 Mishler (1981, 149-51) illustrates how the treatment of a physical condition, a high blood sugar level, is affected by social, structural and cultural factors.

This example suggests that there should be a retraining of those who diagnose and treat illness, in favour of a more holistic approach. According to Bennet (1987, 228-31), there are three mains parts to holistic medicine: (a) the conceptual, (b) the practical and (c) the personal.

> (a) *Conceptual*. The holistic model of illness assumes that the doctor will take account, not only of the body, but of the mind and the spirit as well; and there is a further assumption that everything is interconnected, that all events affect one another, and the organism is in constant interaction with the environment.
>
> (b) *Practical*. From the practical point of view, the holistic practitioner should seek the best treatment available, regardless of the philosophy underlying it. Thus, in practice, holistic medicine would be pragmatic. However, the practical aim of holistic practice is not only to remove symptoms, but to help sick people take stock of their lives . . . and how in the future they can better maintain a balance in their lives.
>
> (c) *Personal*. The ideas and practice of holistic medicine make personal demands on the doctor and the patient in a way which orthodox medicine does not. Both doctor and patient have obligations to live sensibly and not to abuse their systems with harmful foodstuffs or hectic life-styles. Orthodox medicine is engaged in a small way in what is called "health education", but nowhere is any serious attempt made to *oblige* people to look after themselves.
> Reprinted by permission of Martin Secker & Wargburg Ltd.

Box 2.1

THE TREATMENT OF HIGH BLOOD SUGAR LEVELS: MEDICAL THEORY AS A BELIEF SYSTEM

It is not uncommon for a physician to diagnose an illness in a clinically asymptomatic patient when some key biological sign or indicator of the illness is found in a physical examination or laboratory test. One example is an elevated blood sugar level, often used as a principal criterion in the diagnosis of adult-onset diabetes. Nowadays, relatively few adult patients appear in a physician's office with the overt clinical syndrome of diabetes, "characterized by polyphagia, polydipsia, and polyuria, loss of weight and other signs and symptoms attributable to hyperglycemia, glycosuria, and other consequences of a disordered metabolism of carbohydrate fat and protein." The case is different for children, but adults may come to be diagnosed as diabetic when sugar is found in their urine during a routine medical examination. Typically, the finding is unanticipated, because the person has been asymptomatic. Sometimes referred to as "chemical" diabetics or as having "subclinical" diabetes, these patients will then usually be placed on a treatment regimen that may include a special diet, tablets, or insulin injections. The essential aim of the treatment is to reduce blood sugar levels so that they approximate "normal" levels, and thereby prevent development of the clinical symptoms of diabetes listed earlier. It is also believed by some diabetologists that other complications of the disease, such as microvascular disorders, may be diminished or prevented through strict control of blood sugar levels.

Although this approach to the control of adult diabetes is quite widespread, one investigator argues that the grounds for both diagnosis and treatment are not particularly definitive. Posner, an anthropologist whose report is based on observations and interviews in a British diabetic outpatient clinic, cites a number of specialists to the effect that a high blood sugar level by itself is an inadequate index of diabetes. Among the difficulties in evaluating the clinical significance of this index are the following: blood sugar levels are subject to considerable fluctuation, with the amount of variation between successive tests in the same person often as great as variations between people; even high levels require reference to other physiologic systems and metabolic processes for adequate interpretation; finally, a strong correlation has not been established between the severity of diabetes as measured by blood sugar levels and the development of complications.

The efficacy of treatment is also far from being well demonstrated [. . .] In addition, although treatment is prescribed to reduce the risk of complications and symptoms that may result from chronic hyperglycemia, hypoglycemic attacks from taking insulin appear to be more common than the effects of hyperglycemia among adult diabetics under treatment. One of Posner's respondents told her of one survey that reported hypoglycemia as "the most common complication" in long-term diabetic patients. These results suggest that a significant complication of adult-onset diabetes may be iatrogenic, that is, treatment-induced.

On the basis of her study, Posner argues that the evidence is equivocal with regard to the link between high blood sugar levels and the serious sequelae of diabetes. Nonetheless, active treatment with insulin injections or tablets is commonly prescribed, often in conjunction with diet recommendations. Posner then asks why the hypothesis guiding the diagnosis and treatment of diabetes has not been seriously challenged or replaced in clinical practice. She proposes that when physicians are faced with a situation of great uncertainty and the unpredictability of onset of serious and life-threatening complications, it is understandable that they "need to feel that they can at least control it (i.e., blood sugar levels), and that there is something they can do which will help prevent complications." One physician whom she quotes suggests the degree to which the hypothesis' acceptance is a matter of faith: ". . . we all secretly feel that this is in fact the case, . . . we all secretly believe this and hope about it, but there is no outstanding evidence that it is true." Posner concludes that "the medical theory of the treatment of diabetes is a belief system which is sustained by certain medical assumptions and, like any other, by social, structural and cultural factors."

Posner's analyses and interpretation must be qualified in some obvious ways. In particular, she studied only one clinic, and we recognize that there is considerable variation and controversy among diabetologists as to the proper treatment of this complex illness. Nevertheless, [. . .] the biomedical model with its assumption of generic diseases underlies the act of faith she describes, and what she refers to as "magical elements" in clinical practice. Posner points to one set of factors that serves to sustain these practices, namely, the uncertainty and unpredictability of the disease in the context of a physician's commitment to reduce risk and to alleviate suffering. The influence of broader sociocultural values and of the specific definition of physicians' role obligations are evident. For example, there is the general view in medicine that once a technique that can provide some control over a problem is available, it should be used. Thus, when it was found that insulin could reduce blood sugar levels, physicians came to feel that it would be "unethical" not to prescribe it even though it has remained unclear that an elevated blood level is the principal and criterial factor in producing the complications of diabetes.

This example suggests the importance of general social norms and cultural values in the orientation of physicians to their work. They are morally obligated to treat persons who show signs of illness. In the case of diabetes, when an individual is labeled as having this disease on the basis of an elevated blood sugar level, which is a deviation from a biological norm, then treatment of the disease appears to be required by the sociocultural standards of professional practice. [. . .] Thus, although both diagnosis and treatment might appear on the surface to be primarily technical matters, it is clear in this instance that their determinants reflect the sociocultural context of medical practice.

SOURCE: Page 149-51 in E.G. Mishler et al., *Social Contexts of Health, Illness and Patient Care.* Copyright © 1981. Cambridge University Press. Reprinted with the permission of Cambridge University Press.

Before going on to discuss the effects of the social construction of illness/health on the doctor/patient relationship and the medicalization of our society, we need to look at the issue of control as it relates to the concept of health.

The Issue of Control

The recent trend in health discussions concerning the Canadian population tends to focus the blame for illness on the lack of preventive measures taken by the individual (Coreil and Levin 1984-85). The assumption is that illness occurs because of a lack of self-discipline, as in smoking, drinking and eating the wrong foods. The solution is simple: make individuals responsible for their own health. This thinking is exemplified in the Lalonde Report (1981) and the government's "Participaction" program.

It is interesting that 19th-century notions of self-discipline and control of our bodies – notions that valued "character," "well-being," "manhood" and "hard work" – have recurred in the late 20th century.[1] Our perceptions of our ability to be socially productive are linked to these values. In this perspective, health enables us to be economically productive, as well as fulfilled in our daily social relationships. In our culture health care is a very private matter. Our privacy isolates us from each other and reinforces our acceptance of medical knowledge and treatment (Conn and Fox 1980).

However, while people are being urged to exercise self-control, they are being deprived of control over their own health, because of the way medicine is organized in our society. People have begun to react to this loss of control. The women's health movement, for example, is working for women to regain control over their own bodies. The issue of the "right to die" is also part of the struggle to reclaim from medicine our right to our own bodies. The whole patient rights movement is part of the resistance to health-care control. (The issue of patient rights will be dealt with more fully in Chapter 7.)

Loss of control over our own health is due not only to our current medical system; it is also a factor of the way our society is organized. Society makes it hard for us to control the conditions that shape our lives, which are gradually being eroded by the diseases of civilization and destruction of the environment. We might say that the movement for a more holistic medicine is a resistance against our forced participation in an unhealthy society. We can no longer be passive to be healthy, we must actively influence the social conditions we live in.

How much control do the poor have over their health? Rates of infant mortality, and all diseases in general, are higher among the poor and the working class in Canada. Should the blame be placed on them because they lack self-control (they smoke, have bad diets, fail to exercise and drink too much)? These groups often live in poor environments which affect their health, and over which they have little control. For example, the lead content in the air and soil of east-end Toronto and the mercury in the rivers of northern Ontario have a great effect on the lives of people living in these areas.

> Much of the discomfort of modern urban living and not a little of the hazard associated with it, is a direct result of stupid planning, such as thoughtless urban design of roads that run through residential districts where children have no place to play but the street, high-rise apartments that make no concession to the facts of family life when harassed mothers must cope with toddlers on upper floors that have no proper play area. (Last 1982, 378)

Figure 2.1 shows how lead gets into a child's body. In populations affected by this problem, levels of lead in the blood have been reduced not by medical care but by the reduction of lead in gasoline, pipes, cans, etc. (See Golub 1985 for an illustration of the relation between lead in the environment and children's health.) In other words, prevention has been the answer. With this in mind, we need to consider whether public monies should be put into better education and housing for the poor, instead of into medical technology.

We need to be aware that programs which tell us what is "good for us" support a particular view of the world and a particular view of health, which transfers responsibility to the individual. Shifting responsibility from the community, which supports the collective interests of the population, to the individual pits every person against large, well-organized institutions (governments, planners, corporations, etc.). This shift leaves individuals less able to enact changes in their environment and lifestyle. The two sections that follow discuss the doctor/patient relationship and medicalization. Both have to do with the fight between individuals and the medical profession (or the State) over definitions of health and illness.

The Doctor/Patient Relationship

Just as every marriage is actually two marriages, his and hers, so the doctor/patient relationship is experienced quite differently by the two parties involved. Many physicians speak of the sanctity of this relationship, which they see as the hub of medical practice. The physician must inspire confidence in his decisions so that the patient will attempt to follow treatment recommendations. It is within this relationship that the "art" of medicine is practised. The majority of medical decisions made in Canada are made within the context of the doctor/patient relationship.

As patients we surrender to our physicians our most personal information, things we would not tell even our most intimate friends or relations. We also surrender freedom to our bodies. While this freedom and knowledge of our personal lives may be held with reverence by the ideals of the profession, there is evidence that individual physicians do abuse this trust. I am referring not only to the obvious case of sexual assault, but also to the use of patients' bodies in clinical experiments (such as organ transplants). As well, there are practices considered normal by the medical profession that are seen as unnecessary by patients, for

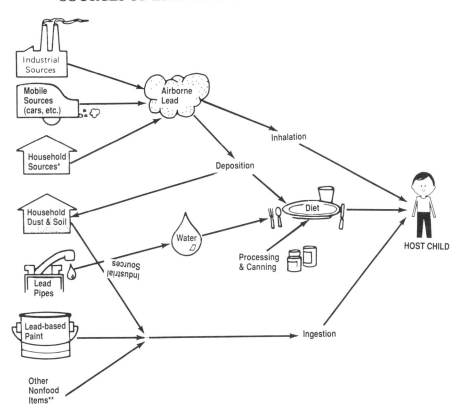

FIGURE 2.1

SOURCES OF LEAD IN A CHILD'S ENVIRONMENT

*Production of bullets or fishing sinkers
  Soldering and stained-glass work
  Gasoline sniffing
  Pottery glazing
  Burning of batteries, colored newsprint, lead-painted objects, and waste oil

**Toys and figures containing lead
  Folk remedies
  Cosmetics (especially Oriental cosmetics, e.g., Surma, a black eyeliner)
  Jewelry (painted with lead to simulate pearl)
  Lead-contained dust transmitted on clothing from workplace.

SOURCE: 1985 Statement "Preventing Lead Poisoning in Children" Centre for Disease Control. Reprinted by permission.

example, asking if a patient is married when discussing contraception, or asking a female patient to disrobe for a routine examination (such as a pap test).

Medical educators (those who teach in medical schools) who do not believe a control/dependence relation should exist between doctor and patient work on ways to improve the interaction between doctor and patient through better communication (Thompson 1984 *inter alia*). It is argued by those who support better communication between doctor and patient that the success of this interaction, and the better health of the patient, depend on the patient's understanding and then obeying the doctor. "Treatment of a disease is clearly inadequate if the patient does not follow the treatment" (Armstrong 1980, 73). Often patients do not follow the treatment: it has been estimated that in Britain almost 20% of all prescriptions are never presented to a pharmacist and about 33% of filled prescriptions are not taken (Armstrong 1980, 73).

While communication between doctor and patient may be crucial (see Braunstein and Silverman 1981), there are serious obstacles to achieving such communication: there are inherent status differences between doctor and patient (Mishler 1984), and the two parties are seeking differing answers to the illness (Helman 1984, 88-92).

Some sociologists claim that the existing structure of the doctor/patient relationship, and its place within social relationships in general, reproduces a particular view of relations of authority, favouring the physicians' opinions, and focuses on issues and solutions (such as getting patients to take their medication) which serve the interests of the profession or dominant groups in the society, and not those of the patient (Borges 1986 *inter alia*). Blind obedience on the part of the patient only creates dependence.

Roles and Rituals

Within the doctor/patient relationship, there are specific roles for the patient and specific roles for the physician which are enforced by the interaction between them (Fisher and Todd 1986). The roles will be described in the models below. As well, certain rituals are carried out. Helman (1984, 87) describes the interaction as containing:

(1) the presentation of "illness" by the patient, both verbally and non-verbally;
(2) the translation of these diffuse symptoms or signs into the named pathological entities of medicine, that is, converting "illness" into "disease"; and
(3) the prescribing of a treatment regimen which is acceptable to both doctor and patient.

Traditional sociologists argue that certain rules and regulations (concerning rituals and roles) exist in the ideal doctor/patient interaction (Parsons 1953) to ensure that the needs of both physician and patient are met. For example, the authority and expertise of the physician is reinforced by the setting of the interaction (hospital, clinic, office) which ensures that the physician will act in a professional manner and that the patient will obey the physician's demands. However, it has been shown that different rules apply to different situations, depending on the patient and the nature of the illness (Szasz and Hollender 1956).

Patients come to the doctor/patient interaction with different goals or expectations than do physicians (Fitzpatrick et al. 1984). We know from the section on clinical practice that the physician enters a discussion with the patient from a particular biomedical context, and that the physician's concern is the elimination of the disease, not the functional health of the patient. Doctors are concerned with their ability to perform, follow their particular routine, and make the patient feel better. Patients' expectations vary greatly; they are not as homogeneous as physicians in regard to education, social class, gender and ethnicity.

The doctor/patient relationship is not one of equality, not one in which the participants are willing to negotiate; there is *inequality* of knowledge and of power (Friedson 1970, 315-21). Mishler (1984) and others (Fisher and Todd 1986) show how the dialogue between the doctor and the patient structures the flow of information and fosters the patient's dependence on the physician. The interview is led by the physician and the definition of relevant information is made by the physician. If the patient wants help from the physician, she must abide by the rules of the interview. The case history in Box 2.2 illustrates just how this process of structuring information and creating dependence occurs.

Box 2.2

THE STRUCTURING OF INFORMATION WITHIN THE DOCTOR/PATIENT RELATIONSHIP

Balint describes the case of Mr. U., aged 35, a skilled workman who was partly disabled due to polio in childhood. Nevertheless he had managed to work, "over-compensating his physical shortcomings by high efficiency". One day he received a severe electric shock at work, and was knocked unconscious; no organic damage was found at the hospital, and he was discharged. He then consulted his family doctor for 'pains' in all parts of his body, which were getting worse and worse: "he thought that something had happened to him through the electric shock". Despite exhaustive tests, no physical abnormality was found, but Mr. U. still experienced his symptoms: "They seem to think I am imagining things: I know what I've got." He still felt definitely "ill" and wanted "to know what condition he could have causing all these pains." Despite more hospital tests that were negative, he still felt himself to be ill. In Balint's view he was "proposing an illness" to the doctor, but this was consistently rejected; the doctor's emphasis was not on the patient's pains, anxieties, fears and hopes for sympathy and understanding, but on the exclusion of an underlying physical abnormality.

SOURCE: C. Helman, *Culture, Health and Illness*. Bristol: John Wright and Sons, 1984. P. 89-90.

A number of questions could be asked about this case. How does it illustrate the interaction between doctor and patient in the clinical setting? What are the needs of each of the participants? Does the power of the physician over diagnosis affect the well-being of the patient? Are there possible solutions to this problem?

Models of the Doctor/Patient Relationship

There are three different models which try to capture the content of the roles and interaction in the doctor/patient relationship. These are: (1) the traditional, (2) the interactive and (3) the structural. The first two are concerned with describing and prescribing how patients and doctors interact; that is, they use the sociology *in* medicine approach. The third model focuses on the effects of the doctor/patient relationship on our perceptions of authority and expert opinion; this model is drawn from the sociology *of* medicine and prescribes a change in the relationship. These three models differ as to which party (doctor or patient) has the right and the ability to make decisions. The point of these models is to develop a guide to studying doctor/patient relations, in order that more research can be done on improving this critical area of health care.

The Traditional Model

The traditional view of the doctor/patient interaction is exemplified in the work of Talcott Parsons (1951 and 1953). In Parsons' model there are specific roles for the participants to play in the clinical interaction. The patient is expected to reveal to the doctor all information concerning her illness. She is expected to trust the doctor and obey his recommendations without question. The doctor, on the other hand, is expected to act in a professional manner, which includes working in the "best interests" of the patient. He is also expected to be objective and emotionally detached, while applying a high degree of skill and knowledge to the problem at hand. This traditional model assumes that physicians are experts and that they will act in the best interests of their patients and of society. In this model the patient is seen as uneducated and passive and thus should be guided to health by an authority. In other words, "Doctor knows best."

A few comments on this model are in order. Many Canadians do not feel comfortable allowing the physician to know every detail of their personal lives. Single parents, people on welfare, homosexuals, and persons having many lovers may not feel they can safely disclose this information to their physician. And the physician might indeed have biases against such people. The personal and political views of physicians are often embedded within their scientific opinions, so that health is linked to morality (Borges 1986, 28).

The Interactive Model

Szasz and Hollender (1956) state that many doctor/patient relationships do not resemble the traditional model described above. In fact they go as far as to say that the Parsonian model is not even desirable. They state that there is no set doctor/patient relationship which will work best for all cases, but instead three basic models which take account of the doctor, the patient and the patient's illness. These models, shown in Table 2.1, differ according to the degree of inequality/equality in the relationship. For example, the physician is less powerful in the mutual participation model than in the activity/passivity model.

TABLE 2.1

THE THREE BASIC INTERACTIVE MODELS OF THE DOCTOR/PATIENT RELATIONSHIP

Model	Physician's Role	Patient's Role	Clinical Application of Model	Prototype of Model
Activity-passivity	Does something to patient	Recipient (unable to respond or inert)	Anesthesia, acute trauma, coma, delirium, etc.	Parent-infant
Guidance-cooperation	Tells patient what to do	Cooperator (obeys)	Acute infectious processes, etc.	Parent-child (adolescent)
Mutual participation	Helps patient to help himself	Participant in "partnership" (uses expert help)	Most chronic illnesses, psychoanalysis, etc.	Adult-adult

SOURCE: T. Szasz and M. Hollender. "The Basic Models of the Doctor-Patient Relationship." *Archives in Internal Medicine* vol. 97 (1956). P. 586. Copyright 1956, American Medical Association.

This model is given validity by the patients' rights movement which is growing in Canada and having a dramatic effect on the doctor/patient relationship. Coburn (1980, 15) says that in the past the health care system has been ". . . run more for the benefit, convenience, and in the interest of those providing care than for the ease and comfort of patients." (Although the interests of those providing health are sometimes the same as those of the patients, often they are different.) The goal of this model is for doctors to become sensitive to their patients' needs, while the patients become more aware of what doctors are doing.

While the doctor wishes to achieve an accurate view of the patient's needs, the patient also wants something from the doctor. Simply making a diagnosis and giving a standardized explanation is often not sufficient for the patient though it may be for the doctor. (Innes 1977, 635)

The Structural Model

The structural model of the doctor/patient relationship places this relationship within the larger social context, without losing sight of the one-on-one interaction between the two parties (Waitzkin 1979; Waitzkin and Stoeckle 1976). After observing a number of doctor/patient relationships, Waitzkin and Stoeckle (1976, 264) made the following comment:

What the doctor told a patient seemed to depend on what kind of person the doctor was, as well as the characteristics of the particular patient. In addition, [we] noticed that the situation in which doctors and patients interact – private practice, outpatient departments, emergency rooms, etc. – seemed to make a difference in the nature of their communication. This variability also seemed to occur for problems that were much less serious than cancer. Some patients with relatively minor disorders seemed to receive little information from their doctors, while other patients obtained more.

In the structural model the context of the interaction is based on the transmission of information from each participant to the other.

In a study on the micro-political relations between doctors and patients, Waitzkin (1979) found that the demystification of medicine, or the education of patients, is crucial in helping patients gain more control over their health care. Patient education is important since it destroys myths about health and enables patients to ask for and obtain information which may add to their ability to make rational decisions about their health, without having to depend on the physician.

Physicians, however, usually do not educate their patients.

. . . The most prevalent form of relationship is one characterized by a dominant and active doctor and a passive and dependent patient. The image of the doctor as health educator freely giving out information is not one which appears to have a realistic basis. This type of relationship may change as a result of the practice of health education in the consultation. However, the structure of the present-day doctor-patient relationship seems to have been produced not just by the substance and the content involved in the consultation but also by the structure of professional-client relations in Western industrial society. Thus, it may not be enough to argue that this problem of patients receiving inadequate information is due to the poor communication skills of the doctor and that this can be remedied by teaching these skills during medical training. (Morgan et al. 1985, 137)

The amount of time doctors spend giving explanations is minimal, and the patient's need for information is often underestimated. This is particularly true in the fee-for-service setting that exists in Canada, whereby physicians are paid according to the particular procedure, rather than according to the amount of time spent. Therefore, the faster doctors accomplish their task, the more money they make. In other words, there is an incentive *not* to spend time educating the patient or explaining complex procedures. When dealing with diseases such as cancer, physicians sometimes choose to be evasive.

By clarifying the verbal and non-verbal behavioural mechanisms (the roles and rituals) which lead to control in doctor/patient relationships "we can begin to reverse the power relationships that [make up] the micropolitics of health care" (Waitzkin 1979, 608).

The Placebo Effect

Many physicians argue that it is not so much the science of medicine that helps people, it is the effect of the patient's belief in the treatment process, or the "placebo effect." The interaction with and the trust in the physician are said by doctors to be the "best medicine." It is generally known in every culture that faith in the curative process is important to its success. In our culture, studies have shown that patients get better from almost every ailment when given a placebo, which is a harmless or inert substance, such as a sugar pill. Rose et al. (1985b, 56-57) argue that since the mind and body are a unity, the reduction of anxiety in the patient through belief in the physician will help the body cure itself. The will of the individual to get well is also essential.

Because of the position of the physician as expert in our society, the physician becomes a generator of the placebo effect. Therefore, the medical argument goes, allowing ourselves to be controlled by the physician, as in the traditional model outlined by Parsons, will aid in the process of healing. This argument is also used as a rationale to withhold information from the patient; that is, if the patient does not know what is wrong, she cannot worry about it.

However, use of this argument by doctors is contradictory, because modern medical practitioners are moving away from emphasis on the emotional or psycho-social aspects of healing.

The New Our Bodies, Ourselves, a guide to women's health care, sees the "art" of medical practice in a different way:

> There may always be something about the "laying on of hands" that calls up the child in us and makes us feel dependent, especially when pain and fear are present. Many physicians deliberately work to increase this natural phenomenon into a special kind of dependency in which the patient turns to the physician for guidance in all kinds of personal problems. (Boston Women's Health Collective 1984, 562)

The authors go on to point out that this dependence response does not just happen. Many medical schools, residency programs and instructors, implicitly and explicitly, teach the techniques of eliciting dependency from patients and maintaining the authority of the physician (Parlow and Robinson 1974, 8-12).

Information Control

One of the most important factors in the relationship between doctor and patient is the exchange of information. The patient's control over her own health is dependent on the amount of information she has. However, information continues to be withheld by physicians or used to mislead the patient.

Control involves the amount of knowledge that patients have about their illness and the willingness of physicians to educate their patients. The technical language of the physician, the misunderstandings around the taking of prescriptions, and the fear and feelings of inadequacy of the patient all add to the friction between doctor and patient. Information control is thus part of the general control over the patient's body.

Pendleton and Bochner (1980) show that various social factors, such as social class and gender, affect the amount of information doctors give to patients. Their research also shows that the ability of physicians to communicate and help patients is not inherent, but must be learned.

Since we all turn to our doctor, as expert, to solve many of our personal as well as our health problems, the physician's power to make decisions about people's lives is great. Too often medical research fails to look at the physician's behaviour and motives. Instead it sees the patient as problematic.

Waitzkin and Stoeckle, who studied interactions between doctors and patients, have stated that ". . . the nature of information transmittal between doctors and patients showed something about society more generally. It seemed to show how some people – that is, experts or professionals – maintain power over other people – clients, patients, etc. – by controlling the information that is communicated" (1976, 264).

Canadian law now upholds the patient's right of access to her own medical record (Rozovsky 1979, 95). Gaining this right was a struggle against the medical profession.

Medicalization

Medicalization is the ". . . bringing of more and more aspects of daily life into the medical sphere of influence" (Doyal 1979, 17). In practical terms this is done by ". . . making medicine and the labels 'healthy' and 'ill' relevant to an ever increasing part of human existence" (Zola 1972, 487). Medicalization is not simply the definition of certain behaviours as sick, but the provision of explanations, remedies, professionals and institutions to support those definitions.

More and more of our behaviour is being defined by medicine.

Medical science assumes the role of societal expert in the systemic explanation of maladapted behaviour: ". . . medical involvement in social problems leads to their removal from religious and legal scrutiny and thus from moral and punitive consequences . . . the problems are placed under medical and scientific scrutiny and thus in objective and therapeutic circumstances" (Zola 1972, 489). For example, if violence is categorized as a medical, instead of a social, problem, then the solution must be medical. Yet violent behaviour is not caused genetically or by a disease invading the body. Therefore, researchers are faced with the problem of what violence is, and who should be cured. In Britain, drugs are being given to sexual offenders to keep them from committing sex crimes. Such offenders are offered a reduced prison term if they will accept the drug. However, most researchers who study sex crimes know that these crimes have less to do with sex than with domination. If we accept the use of drugs for sex offenders, will we begin to see the development of drugs to control every form of behaviour thought to be abnormal by those in positions of authority? Yes, it does sound like *Brave New World.*

Medicalization is seen too in the increasing use of over-the-counter drugs. Lexchin (1984) says that because of easy access to medication and medical healers, we are slowly becoming addicted to the idea of the instant cure. Physicians and researchers as well as the rest of the population expect a drug cure for every ailment. It is well known that physicians readily prescribe tranquillizers to women, including teenagers, to remedy the pains of everyday life, especially depression. This contributes to drug reliance, which in turn is a factor in the increasing rates of drug overdoses among this population.

There is a relation between the pressure on physicians from drug companies to use drug therapy and physicians' willingness to rely on such treatment. Doctors' magazines abound in glossy drug advertisements. In 1978, approximately $290,000 per physician was spent annually by drug companies on advertising in Canada. Today the amount is even higher (Lexchin 1984, 112). According to Canadian government statistics,

> . . . 41% of men and 55% of women use drugs. Nearly 60% of boys under five years consume drugs; however, this proportion decreases until age 45, by which time it has dropped to 49%. At the age of 65 and over, 66% of men use drugs. A similar pattern prevails among women; yet, towards the age of 20 the portion of drug consumers begins to rise, reaching 77% among women aged 65 and over. (Lapierre 1984, 29)

Physicians claim, in their own defence, that their patients pressure them for an instant cure or remedy. Yet physicians perpetuate this situation by not informing their patients when there is little that can be done. The rationale is that anything the doctor does will help, through the placebo effect. (Even drug companies acknowledge that placebos account for about 30% of all recoveries.) Many have even predicted that we are headed for a "therapeutic state," in which all our cares would be eliminated with drugs and in which physicians would be the ministers.

Many physicians say that we should have regular, yearly check-ups. For certain procedures and certain groups this may be beneficial (for example, women benefit by having yearly pap smears). But there is no evidence that regular, annual visits to a physician prolong life. What is the role of medicine today: is it the curing of disease or the buffering of the pains of everyday life? Probably the latter is true, more and more.

We have come to a point in history where most of the traditional means of dealing with illness and death have been eliminated and our health has become directly related to our ability to survive as a society. Many experts say that we have reached a plateau in health care and that our life expectancy and rates of morbidity and mortality cannot be changed by the type of medical system we have today. Perhaps some pain is a normal part of life and must be accepted. We must think seriously about the effect of increasing medical intrusion in our lives. and whether medicine is creating a healthier society. What is the connection between our social relations and the need to be healthy? What part do we ourselves play in the decisions about our health care? We cannot just sit back passively and wait for medicine to cure us.

Childbirth

Childbirth is a good example of the process of medicalization (Leavitt 1986, Oakley 1984). In earlier times, medicine had little or nothing to do with childbirth. Since the early 20th century there has been a growing conflict between the medical profession and women who want to have their babies outside the hospital setting. This can be seen today in the disputes over the provincial legalization of midwifery and the facilitation of home births. The question to be asked is, since there is nothing "sick" about giving birth, why is medicine involved, and why is there such a strong reaction by the medical profession against the reinstatement of midwifery as an independent, non-medical profession.[2]

> Midwives disappeared first from urban Ontario around the turn of the century. In British Columbia and the Yukon, there never were very many. The last significant generation of Prairie midwives probably apprenticed during the Depression decade. An elderly Quebecoise midwife recalls that in 1942, her license was simply not renewed. In the Maritimes midwives worked for a time in cooperation with home birth doctors, until the road system improved and birth moved into the hospitals. Only in Newfoundland [. . .] did midwifery survive as a province-wide institution as late as the 1960's. (Barrington 1985, 29)

The survival of midwifery in Newfoundland is probably due to that province's attachment to Britain, where medical and lay midwifery is well organized.

Those who argue for home births say that, for a normal birth, a home is a safer place than a hospital, both physically and emotionally. Home births are the norm in other countries.

In Holland, 70 percent of all births still take place in the home, with no apparent influence on infant or maternal mortality statistics. In our society, the woman in labour is rushed to the hospital, where an array of trained strangers are responsible for guiding her through the experiences of birth and initial care of the newborn. (Mumford 1983, 165)

The argument by the Canadian Medical Association (CMA) is that, because of the possibility of complications, it is better for childbirth to take place in a hospital under the surveillance of the medical profession, where technology is available. The rule of medical control is thus enforced because of a minority of cases, and childbirth, which is not an illness, is drawn into the scope of medical expertise and treatment. There is a spiralling of technology: the use of medical intervention promotes the use of more medical intervention. As Barrington shows (see Table 2.2), the chain of events in childbirth is distorted by medical intervention, and this intervention in a number of cases actually causes a health risk to mother and child.

Women who demand a hospital birth may do so out of fear for the safety of the child and their own life. However the data available do not show that home births are unsafe. In countries where midwifery is legal or where traditional methods of birth are used, home birth is the norm. Rates of infant mortality in some of these countries are equal to or even lower than those in Canada. Even within Canada there are great differences in the infant mortality rate according to geographic area and ethnic group. For example the infant mortality rate for Canada as a whole in 1961 was 27.3, and in 1971 it was 17.5. However, for the Northwest Territories in 1961 it was 111.0, and in 1971 it was 49.0 (Manitoba 1975, 47). Further figures on infant mortality in Canada are given in Table 2.3.

A recent study (Ohlsson and Fohlin 1983) comparing infant care in Sweden and Ontario shows that prenatal health care of the mother has a great effect on decreasing **perinatal mortality**. This study, along with evidence on reduced mortality from countries with organized midwives, shows the importance of a total birthing system, covering the time from conception to the child's first birthday. In countries with high infant mortality rates, the lowering of these rates will be brought about more by better food, water and housing than by medical practice (McKeown 1979).

The way in which health care is organized and focused may affect the rates of specific types of infant mortality (Ohlsson and Fohlin 1983). For example, from 1969 to 1980, **post-neonatal** deaths (4 weeks to a year) rose, while **neonatal** deaths (under 28 days) decreased (Canada 1983c,

TABLE 2.2

CHAIN OF EVENTS DISTORTING CHILDBIRTH

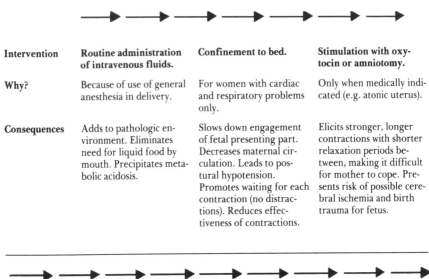

Intervention	Routine administration of intravenous fluids.	Confinement to bed.	Stimulation with oxytocin or amniotomy.
Why?	Because of use of general anesthesia in delivery.	For women with cardiac and respiratory problems only.	Only when medically indicated (e.g. atonic uterus).
Consequences	Adds to pathologic environment. Eliminates need for liquid food by mouth. Precipitates metabolic acidosis.	Slows down engagement of fetal presenting part. Decreases maternal circulation. Leads to postural hypotension. Promotes waiting for each contraction (no distractions). Reduces effectiveness of contractions.	Elicits stronger, longer contractions with shorter relaxation periods between, making it difficult for mother to cope. Presents risk of possible cerebral ischemia and birth trauma for fetus.

Use of analgesics anesthesia.	Use of forceps.	Supine-Lithotomy position.	Episiotomy.
Substituted for emotional support from family. Used when medically indicated (e.g. prolonged labor).	For complicated or arrested second stage of labor.	Convenience for active management of birth by obstetrician.	Result of developing a table with stirrups and using forceps for delivery. Lack of patience in waiting out the course of labor and of training in basic measures to comfort women and facilitate second stage of labor.
Produces lethargic mother who is unable to respond actively to the labor process and narcotized infant with possible respiratory and neurological complications.	Necessitates lithotomy position and episiotomy. May lead to possible damage of infant's facial nerve or brachial plexus or intracranial hemorrhage.	Requires mother to move at difficult time from labor room to delivery room table. Inhibits mother's voluntary efforts to expel infant. Increases tension of perinatal tissues. May lead to supine hypotension with resulting decrease of oxygen to fetus.	Requires strapping mother to table and shaving perineum to maintain sterile field. Necessitates at least local anesthesia. Initiates painful postpartum recuperation, thus leading to more pain medication.

SOURCE: E. Barrington, *Midwifery is Catching.* Toronto: NC Press, 1985. P. 129.

TABLE 2.3

INFANT DEATHS, INFANT MORTALITY RATE AND AGE-SPECIFIC DISTRIBUTION OF INFANT DEATHS, CANADA, 1931, 1956 AND 1981

| | Infant deaths | | Percentage distribution of deaths by age | | | |
Year	Number	Rate[1]	Less than 7 days	7-27 days	28 days and over	Total
1931[2]	20,360	86.0[3]	34.1	14.6	51.4	100.0
1956	14,399	31.9	52.3	10.7	37.0	100.0
1981	3,562	9.6	57.2	9.0	33.8	100.0

SOURCE: Y. Peron and C. Strohmenger, *Demographic and Health Indicators*. Ottawa: Statistics Canada, 1985. P. 195. Reproduced with permission.

[1] Per 1,000 live births.
[2] Excluding Newfoundland, Yukon and Northwest Territories.
[3] Including Newfoundland, Yukon and Northwest Territories.

23). These rates may be affected by our recent focus on saving a child's life at birth.

> . . . mortality during the neonatal period is being shifted to the post neo-natal period as a result of medical breakthroughs that are prolonging the lives of infants born with severe handicaps. (Dumas 1984, 24)

However, our ability to keep children alive at very low birth weights has caused an increase in the number of handicapped children. The remedies used to keep children alive often result in problems after birth. Yet there is little being done about the increased demand for social services by the families of these handicapped children. (Not only the medical profession but the general population as well must realize that not every child that is born will be perfect, and some children will die.)

In relation to childbirth there is a growing medical concern for economic efficiency and the physician's personal schedule.[3] These factors, in addition to financial cutbacks and the reduced amount of time the physician has to spend with each patient, may account for the growing cases of induced labour and caesarean births (Martin et al. 1982): in Quebec caesarean sections increased from 6.8% of all births in 1971 to 17.6% in 1983-1984. These statistics can be seen as a phenomenon of the system of medicalization, which could be changed by a better organization of health care. It has always been assumed that a woman who has had one caesarean birth must have all subsequent children that way, but there is no evidence to support this assumption.

In some cases caesarean operations may be necessary to save the life of the mother and child, but in other cases they are unnecessary and even harmful. "Cesarian section is still a major operation and the procedure is associated with substantial maternal morbidity" (Martin et al. 1982, 85). However, the medical profession now regards the caesarean as a standard procedure.

Another example: studies show that 68.9% of Quebec women giving birth were given **episiotomies** in 1983-1984. Again, there is no evidence to show that this procedure has any advantage in the typical birth, and may in fact cause sexual problems for the woman after birth. It may simply be a way for doctors to hasten the birth process.

> The medical domination of the process of pregnancy and childbirth has produced growing disquiet. On the one hand, there is a growing demand for women to be able to choose to have their babies at home where there are no medical indications of the necessity for a hospital delivery. On the other hand, there is a growing criticism of the unnecessary and demeaning rituals which are involved in hospital deliveries – the shaving of pubic hair for example. . . . In recent years, these criticisms have concentrated to a considerable extent on what has been called the "active management of labour", and particularly on the increase in the number of induced births. (Doyal 1979, 235)

The argument for the de-medicalization of childbirth and the reinstatement of midwifery is strengthened when we consider the number of cases of illness in the mother and child caused by hospitalization.[4] After all, the hospital is a centre of disease. "Hospital acquired infections are an increasingly common clinical and epidemiological problem" (Randall 1980, 119). The rates of **nosocomial** (hospital-acquired) infections ranges from 4% to 10% of all patients entering Canadian hospitals.

> Patients entering hospital and other health institutions are at considerable risk of acquiring an infection. They have an underlying medical condition and possibly are also on medication which may compromise their ability to resist infection. They enter an environment where they must be subjected to diagnostic and therapeutic instrumentation and medication, where other patients may harbour organisms in direct proximity, and where microorganisms often evolve into antibiotic resistant subtypes. (Losos and Totman 1984, 248)

A woman entering a hospital to give birth becomes part of a **population at risk** of contracting a **virus** or **bacteria** which may cause illness or even death. Clare Randall (1980, 119) cites an outbreak of pseudomonas cepacia (a bacterium) in the Victoria Hospital in London, Ontario, that had been caused by contaminated distilled water in the pharmacy. Outbreaks of infections in hospitals are in fact more common than thought (Belle et al. 1979). Some of the ways in which these infections are transmitted are through contaminated topical solutions, commercially packaged catheter kits, and contaminated distilled water.

Although it is illegal (as of 1988) for midwives to practise in most Canadian provinces, governments are beginning to favour the midwife. In 1987 the Ontario government started a plan to integrate nurse-midwifery into the medical system. This recent change of heart may be explained in economic terms: the cost of the midwife in relation to the physician is quite low, and hospitalization for childbirth is a substantial part of total hospital costs. In 1977, "childbirth was the major reason for hospitalization of women (17% of the cases)" (Lapierre 1984, 31). Childbirth accounts for approximately 70% of all hospital use for women aged 20 to 44. In Manitoba, the highest cost per patient was in the category of pregnancy and childbirth (Manitoba 1984, 34).

A few members of the medical profession have realized that midwifery is a vital link in the system of health and care and are therefore leaning toward its reinstatement (Barrington 1985). However, if midwives are once more allowed to practise, it will be under the control of the medical profession; they will not be allowed to become an independent health **profession** or practise outside the control of the physician. This restriction is already happening in Ontario. Furthermore, physicians will become specialists in midwifery.

To conclude this section on childbirth, midwifery will be legalized, but unfortunately it will also be medicalized. It should have been possible to have the legalization without medicalization.

Iatrogenic Illness

Iatrogenic illness, or **iatrogenesis**, is illness caused by medical treatment. We have reached a point at which scientific medicine can do little to change the major causes of death, but has increased the amount of physician-induced illness. Illich (1976) and others have shown that medicine and hospitals create more illness, disease and suffering than they eliminate.

> One in fifty children admitted to a hospital suffers an accident which requires specific treatment. University hospitals are relatively more pathogenic, or, in blunt language, more sickening. It has also been established that one out of every five patients admitted to a typical research hospital acquires an iatrogenic disease, sometimes trivial, usually requiring special treatment, and one case in thirty leading to death. Half of these episodes result from complications of drug therapy; amazingly, one in ten comes from diagnostic procedures. (Illich 1976, 32)

Medically induced illness is a problem since approximately one out of every six Canadians will enter a hospital for treatment this year and one out of every two Canadians will visit an outpatient centre, emergency room or clinic.

> The history of medicine is replete with examples of illness resulting from sound therapeutic endeavour. The emergence of a new syndrome while the patient is being

treated for another condition has long been recognized in clinical medicine. However, in recent years the development of potent new therapeutic agents, improved surgical procedure and more efficient equipment has forced this facet of medicine into unprecedented prominence. (Moser 1956, 606)

Ivan Illich (1976) sees three categories of iatrogenic illness: clinical, social and cultural. *Clinical* iatrogenesis is damage done to a person's health by the application of medication by physicians. Many drugs have side effects. Physicians are only beginning to understand the adverse reactions individuals can have to **antibiotics**, and how the overuse of these drugs can lead to their ineffectiveness and to the development of new strains of bacteria (Mumford 1983, 464). Other, starker examples of drugs and treatments that proved harmful include thalidomide and DES, discussed earlier, Depo-Provera, which has produced deformed children and sterility in women (Green 1987), and the Dalkon Shield. Clinical iatrogenesis would also include the prolonging of suffering by keeping people alive. Nosocomial (hospital-induced) infections are a third example of clinical iatrogenesis. *Social* iatrogenesis is the loss of control over our own health. People submit their bodies to the bureaucracy of medicine, yet are eliminated from discussions and decisions about treatment. Thus, the powerful medical profession alienates us from our bodies. *Cultural* iatrogenesis is the elimination from our culture of the means, rituals, and values that would enable us to deal with suffering, death and other unpleasant facts of life. (For the treatment of these in other cultures, see Bloch and Parry 1982.)

Other writers back up Illich's view of the potential harm caused by medicine. "There is growing evidence that many medical products and techniques, including a variety of common surgical procedures and a considerable number of drugs, have little or no efficacy. More seriously, it is becoming increasingly clear that certain medical procedures are not merely ineffective but positively harmful and many themselves cause damage to health" (Doyal 1979, 292-93).

Topliss (1978, 186-88) states:

It is, of course, arguable that where medicalization of a normal process has led to less discomfort and better survival, the process has been justified. Illich, however, stresses the unnecessary treatments imposed on people experiencing normal processes, which can sometimes cause or increase discomfort, or even jeopardize health.

Medicine and the Social Order

Medicalization is closely related to the social order. We know that medicalization is a ". . . process of expansion by which more and more areas of life become subject to medical definition and jurisdiction" (Hillier 1982a, 178-179). This process can be seen as positive or negative, depending on the point of view taken. Also, it may be positive or negative depending on its effect on particular groups of individuals who receive medical treatment instead of legal punishment, as in the case of deviant and criminal behaviour.

Ehrenreich and Ehrenreich (1978) and Zola (1972) explain the way in which medicalization reinforces a given social order. "It [the institution of medicine] has the power to instill order in society, to inhibit disorder or fundamental change" (Hillier 1982a, 175). In other words, the mediators of medical knowledge (doctors) ensure that the beliefs, values and norms of the society are supported by the act of medical care. This does not mean that doctors are *consciously* out to control our behaviour, and we can assume that they act in ways they perceive to be good for the patient.

Parsons (1953) states that the social order works for the good of all; he does not see any particular group interests as being favoured over others. He says that if the order and stability of society are to be maintained, then the behaviour of the members of that society must be controlled. Included among the members of society are physicians, who act in the interests of the social whole.

According to Durkheim, however, ". . . relationships alone cannot form the basis of a stable social order" since rules and regulations perpetuate certain social solutions which favour one particular group over another (Zeitlin 1984, 90). Navarro (1976) and McKinley (1984) state that medicine is acting in the interests of specific powerful groups (the capitalist class) in the society.

It can be argued that specific professional and social interests are at stake in medicalization: to be precise, medicalization serves the interests of the medical profession. Thus, a given treatment may serve the interests of the profession more than those of the patient, although the profession will claim to be serving (and may believe it is serving) the interests of the patient.

Who defines the patient's interests? In a situation of unequal power (e.g. the doctor/patient relationship), the more powerful party defines the interests of the other. The question then is to what extent patients will be able to influence the practice of medicine.

The term "medical order" refers to the way medicine is organized as a whole made up of interconnected parts. Ehrenreich and Ehrenreich (1978, 48-52) see two types of medical order as existing in our society: disciplinary and cooptative. Disciplinary order is exerted by placing barriers in front of those who wish to gain access to the medical system. It discourages any attempt to become ill, to take on the sick role and remove oneself from family and work responsibilities.

Company doctors have been seen as a major obstacle standing between workers and their right to receive compensation and they have earned the mistrust and scorn of workers. In a number of ways they have questioned workers' eligibility for compensation. They have encouraged strategies to interfere with the processing of claims, appeared on behalf of their companies in appeals of Workers' Compensation Board decisions which favoured workers, and argued that workers' personal lives – smoking, loud music, drinking, sports, etc. – are responsible for their illness, rather than occupational hazards. Despite doctors' claims of neutrality and minimum involvement in compensation cases, evidence suggests that many company doctors continue to protect their employers' interests with regard to compensation. (Walters 1985, 71)

This type of order limits the use of medicine in controlling environmental and workplace hazards.

Cooptative order, on the other hand, expands the use of the medical system. "Such services encourage people both to enter sick roles and to seek professional help in a variety of nonsick situations (for preventive care, contraceptive services, marital difficulties, etc.)." In this type of order, more and more behaviour, or social problems, are defined as sickness or disease. This redefinition expands the area of expertise of the physician. The result is to increase dependency on physicians. Both types of medical order are intermingled in the definitions of health placed upon individual behaviour.

Summary

In summary, the present-day lay conceptions of illness and disease are embedded in our social reality. Even though illness is an individual experience it is conceived of in terms of medicine and our relationship to doctors. "The patient's conception of his illness is also a conception of his relationship to others and to society. Discourse about illness conveys a message about the whole society" (Herzlich and Pierret 1985, 150).

> Although disease is nowadays in the hands of medical science . . . medicine, as an institution, a practice and a body of knowledge, is not independent of collective discourse during a given period in a given society, including our own.

The main points of this chapter are: (1) the definitions of health and illness are constructed as part of a socially interactive system; (2) individuals cannot be held totally responsible for their own health; (3) improvements in health can best be effected through the practice of preventive health care, instead of the current "after-the-fact" medicine; (4) the relationship between doctor and patient contains many roles and rituals to be followed; (5) an individual's recovery from an illness can be affected by what he or she thinks of the ability of medicine to cure the illness; (6) the information which passes between doctor and patient is critical to the process of medical diagnosis and to the patient's health; and (7) medicalization, iatrogenesis and social control are all features of our present system of medicine.

Notes

1. For a history of the concept of the healthy body, see Haley 1978.

2. In Canada today midwives can receive training at Memorial University in Newfoundland and at the University of Alberta, which offers a master's program in Nurse-Midwifery. Those trained for midwifery in Canada practise in the North or in developing countries.

3. There is evidence to suggest that some physicians rush births to avoid being called to the hospital on their weekends off. Other physicians charge their patients extra to be present at the birth.

4. A U.S. study (Steel et al. 1981, 638) found that ". . . 36 percent of 815 consecutive patients on a general medical service of a university hospital had an iatrogenic illness." The authors of *The New Our Bodies, Ourselves* point out that, ". . . in large nurseries, infants receive intermittent and often impersonal care, a poor substitute for mothering. Some nurseries breed Staphylococcus aureus, Streptococcus and Salmonella. These clearly iatrogenic illnesses can be serious, sometimes resulting in infant death" (Boston Women's Health Collective 1984, 377).

Chapter 3

Demography and Epidemiology

In order to get a picture of the health of the Canadian population, we first have to know its structure. We should be familiar with two areas of research: (1) **demography** and (2) **epidemiology**. In general, demography is the study of population. It is concerned with rates, relations, percentages, movements of people, and the aggregation of individuals by social category. Epidemiology, which is the study of **morbidity** or rates of disease, builds on demography and uses demographic materials as a basis for investigation.

> In its broadest sense, demography is the branch of the social sciences that studies the size, characteristics, and distribution of populations in an attempt to understand their patterns. In its broadest sense, epidemiology is the branch of medicine that studies the size, characteristics, and distribution of diseases in an attempt to understand their patterns. (Kurtz and Chalfant 1984, 29)

In the study of epidemiology, both medicine and sociology look at the distribution of a specific variable, disease. This approach is different from that of clinical medicine:

> *Clinical medicine* focusses largely on the medical care of individuals. Typically, these have been sick people who have presented themselves for help; in recent years examination of apparently well people has been encouraged in order to detect disease in early stages. In *population medicine* the community replaces the individual patient as the primary focus of concern. The problem here is to evaluate the health of a defined community, including those members who would benefit from, but do not seek, medical care. (Mausner and Kramer 1985, 2)

Demography gives us a means of understanding changes in the population over time. There is continual creation (birth) and continual destruction (death) of members of the population.[1] Since every population can be broken into different age groups, the size of these **cohorts** will affect the organization of the population as a whole (Ryder 1964). Table 3.1 shows a picture of the Canadian population at six different points in this century.

TABLE 3.1

PERCENTAGE DISTRIBUTION OF THE CANADIAN
POPULATION BY FIVE-YEAR AGE GROUPS
AT TWENTY-YEAR INTERVALS, 1901-1981

Age Group	1901	1921	1941	1961	1981
0-4	12.0	12.0	9.2	12.4	7.3
5-9	11.5	12.0	9.2	11.4	7.3
10-14	10.8	10.4	9.7	10.2	7.9
15-19	10.4	9.2	9.9	7.9	9.5
20-24	9.5	8.0	9.0	6.5	9.6
25-29	7.9	7.8	8.4	6.6	8.9
30-34	6.8	7.4	7.3	7.0	8.4
35-39	6.2	7.2	6.6	7.0	6.7
40-44	5.4	6.0	5.9	6.1	5.5
45-49	4.5	5.0	5.5	5.6	5.2
50-54	3.8	4.1	5.1	4.7	5.1
55-59	3.0	3.2	4.4	3.9	4.8
60-64	2.6	2.7	3.4	3.2	4.0
65-69	2.0	2.0	2.6	2.7	3.5
70+	3.1	2.8	4.1	5.0	6.2

SOURCE: *Census of Canada 1961*, column 1, part 2; *Census of Canada 1981*, table 2. Ottawa: Statistics Canada. Reproduced with permission of the Minister of Supply and Services Canada.

This chapter will first give a picture of the Canadian population and then discuss its health. An introduction to demographic and epidemiological methods will form a basis for understanding health and illness in Canada. The following section will deal with the size of the Canadian population, and with the demographic concepts of fertility, mortality and migration.

The Population of Canada

A population is simply the adding up of all persons inhabiting a specific country, province or city. On 1 June 1986 the population of Canada was 25,588,300 (Canada 1987, 39). This figure is estimated from census records and from the current birth, death and migration rates.[2] Table 3.2 gives the distribution of the Canadian population by province, for 1986. Table 3.3 shows the breakdown of the population by urban and rural dwellers, for 1981.

TABLE 3.2

CANADIAN POPULATION DISTRIBUTION BY PROVINCE, 1986

	Population
Canada	25,354,064
Newfoundland	568,349
Prince Edward Island	126,646
Nova Scotia	873,199
New Brunswick	710,422
Quebec	6,540,276
Ontario	9,133,515
Manitoba	1,071,232
Saskatchewan	1,010,198
Alberta	2,375,278
British Columbia	2,889,207
Yukon	23,504
Northwest Territories	52,238

SOURCE: *Census of Canada 1986.* Ottawa: Statistics Canada. Reproduced with permission of the Minister of Supply and Services Canada.

TABLE 3.3

POPULATION DISTRIBUTION OF URBAN AND RURAL DWELLERS, BY PROVINCE, 1981

	Urban		Rural	
	Over 500,000	Less Than 30,000	Rural Non-Farm	Rural Farm
Canada	41.2	15.8	20.0	4.3
Newfoundland	–	39.3	41.0	.3
Prince Edward Island	–	36.3	53.9	9.8
Nova Scotia	–	24.8	42.8	2.1
New Brunswick	–	20.5	47.1	2.2
Quebec	51.6	14.3	19.5	2.9
Ontario	44.3	13.0	15.1	3.2
Manitoba	54.9	12.7	19.4	9.4
Saskatchewan	–	18.6	23.2	18.6
Alberta	53.1	16.2	14.3	8.5
British Columbia	41.6	17.3	19.9	2.2
Yukon	–	64.0	36.0	–
Northwest Territories	–	48.0	52.0	–

SOURCE: *Census of Canada 1981.* Ottawa: Statistics Canada. Reproduced with permission of the Minister of Supply and Services Canada.

Different areas of the country have different rates of growth. Depending on the focus of health research, it may be important to look at local or provincial rates instead of general rates for the country as a whole. Table 3.4 shows the annual rate of population growth for the different regions of Canada.

TABLE 3.4
ANNUAL RATE OF GROWTH (AS A PERCENTAGE), CANADA, 1981-1983

	1981-1982	1982-1983
East	0.4	1.1
Central	0.9	0.9
West	2.1	1.3
North	2.9	-0.4
Canada	1.2	1.0

SOURCE: J. Dumas, *Current Demographic Analysis*. Ottawa: Statistics Canada, 1984. P. 31.

To graphically display a population, demographers have developed the *population pyramid*, which shows the size of each age group in relation to other groups and to the whole population.

> A population pyramid graphically displays a population's age and sex composition. By showing numbers or proportions of males and females in each age group, the pyramid gives a vivid "picture" of the population's characteristics. The sum of all the age-sex groups in the population equals 100 percent of the population. (Haupt and Kane 1985, 13)

Figure 3.1 shows the age pyramid of the Canadian population for June 1, 1983. Each horizontal bar represents the size of an age group or cohort; males are on the left of the centre line and females are on the right. Age is organized from bottom (0) to top (90+), with year of birth listed on the side. As each cohort (age group) gets older it also gets smaller, because mortality increases with age. The decline in size of a cohort accelerates after the age of 45, so that the pyramid rises to a peak for the oldest cohorts.

The following pages discuss the Canadian population according to the demographic concepts of age, sex, fertility (additions to the population), mortality (subtractions from the population), and migration (movement in and out). The size and structure of the population give an indication of future demands on the health-care system.

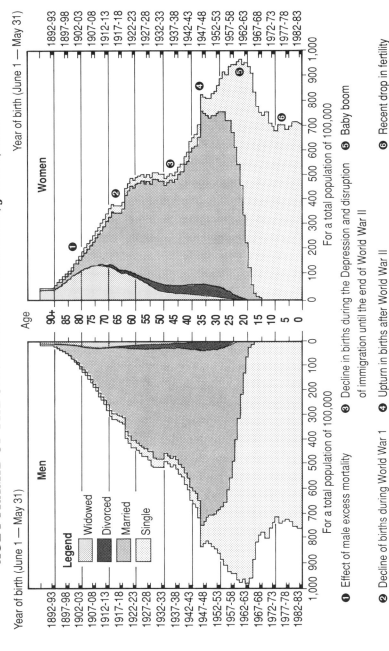

FIGURE 3.1

AGE PYRAMID OF THE CANADIAN POPULATION, JUNE 1, 1983

Legend

- Widowed
- Divorced
- Married
- Single

❶ Effect of male excess mortality

❷ Decline of births during World War 1

❸ Decline in births during the Depression and disruption of immigration until the end of World War II

❹ Upturn in births after World War II

❺ Baby boom

❻ Recent drop in fertility

SOURCE: J. Dumas, *Current Demographic Analysis*. Ottawa: Statistics Canada, 1984. P. 38. Catalogue 91-209E. Reproduced with permission of the Minister of Supply and Services Canada.

Age

Canada, like most developed nations, has an aging population.[3] In 1951 there were 20 people over 65 for every 100 young; in 1983 there were 37 people over 65 for every 100 young.

> The growth in the number of elderly people does not in itself constitute an aging of the population. It is rather their increasing proportion of the population. . . . The elderly segment of the Canadian population will grow proportionately large over the coming decades. (Dumas 1984, 39)

Table 3.5 shows that the proportion of the population 65 and over is growing and will continue to grow in the future.

TABLE 3.5

PERCENTAGE OF THE CANADIAN POPULATION OVER 65, 1901-2051

	% Over 65
1901	5.0
1911	4.7
1921	4.8
1931	5.6
1941	6.7
1951	7.8
1961	7.6
1971	8.1
1981	9.7
1991	11.1*
2001	12.0*
2051	18.2*

SOURCE: Adapted from Tables 1 and 2 in *65 and Older*. Report by National Council of Welfare on Incomes of Aged. National Council of Welfare (1984). P. 31. Reproduced with permission of the Minister of Supply and Services Canada

*Indicates projections.

Knowing the age composition of the population is critical, since changes in this composition will affect the health-care system and health-care costs. By analyzing the population structure and the rate of growth, we can predict the future age structure of the population and the possible needs that will have to be met by the health-care system. Most projections are based on the assumption that present patterns will continue; however we must bear in mind that dramatic changes in the population could occur through war, plague, extremely high or low birth rates, or extremely high immigration or emigration rates.

We know that as people get older they put more demands on the health-care system. Chronic diseases, which are most common among the elderly, increase the length of stay of patients in the hospital and also the possibility of medical intervention and medical cost. However, if the ways of treating chronic disease were to change, the type of care needed by the aged in the future may also change.

There is also the fact that use of the medical system by the elderly is being promoted by medicine itself:

> ... the process of dying provides a very extensive field for potential intervention. Rather than health care utilization being driven by "needs" associated with an aging population, it may be that developments on the supply side, technology and man-power pressures, are driving up use among the elderly. (Evans 1984, 309-310)

In the future, the provincial governments may develop alternative care facilities for the aged, outside hospitals. Nevertheless, there will be growing numbers of elderly in acute care hospitals and concomitant financial strains. One possible development in the future is the introduction of a user fee for those staying in hospital beyond a certain number of days or weeks. This fee would place health costs on the family or the individual and further divide the rich from the poor. The expulsion of the chronically ill elderly from hospitals would have a dramatic effect on health-care costs, since this group is the major user of hospital beds (McDaniel 1986, 81-85).

TABLE 3.6

HOSPITALIZATION BY AGE, CANADA, 1980-1981

	0-14	15-25	25-44	45-64	65+
Separations* per 100,000 population	9,318	12,019	13,531	16,397	34,224
Average length of stay (in days)	5.5	5.9	7.1	12.4	25.8

SOURCE: Adapted from *Hospital Morbidity, 1979-1980 and 1980-1981*. Ottawa: Statistics Canada, 1984. P. 39.
*Separation is the discharge or death of a patient.

Thus, the aging of the population will dramatically affect health care and health-care costs in the future. We can assume that there will be a strain on our existing facilities for chronic care in the future, unless there is an improvement in those facilities or patterns of use (Chappell et al. 1986). To avoid being locked into the present hospital-based system of chronic care, we must look for alternatives to this type of care, while taking account of the social effects of change in the type and place of care.

Sex

The sex **ratio** is expressed as the number of males for every 100 females in the population. The sex ratio at birth is usually 105 or 106 males per 100 females. After birth, however, the sex ratio changes because of mortality and migration. The sex ratio can be calculated for different age cohorts in the population. The population pyramid gives a rough approximation of the sex ratio of the different cohorts.

It is useful to know the sex ratio of the population, since males and females have differing rates of specific diseases. For example, women have higher rates of cerebrovascular diseases and lower rates of respiratory diseases than men have. It is important that the development of health-care facilities take account of these differing needs. An important factor is the willingness of the government to support care and research.[4]

Fertility

In demography, fertility refers to the reproduction of the population, that is, the number of live births and the frequency of births in different social groups. Fertility is affected by **fecundity**, which is the physiological capacity to reproduce (usually applied to women between the ages 15-44), economic development, the age structure, marriage and cohabitation patterns and other factors. In other words, fertility is affected not only by physiology, but also by sociological factors. Since Canadians are tending to have smaller families and are postponing having their first child, the trend to a decrease in fertility is bound to continue.

The decline in the Canadian fertility rate is significant, since at a certain point the population will cease to reproduce itself and will begin dying out. There are voluntary and involuntary reasons for this decline. Voluntary reasons are those which the individual and society can adjust; they will vary over time. Involuntary reasons are those over which we have little control and which have resulted with the development of our civilization.

Voluntary reasons include:

(1) the advantages of a smaller family size (economic and social);
(2) cultural or moral restrictions on marital and sexual relations;
(3) the development of contraception; and
(4) the availability of abortion.

Involuntary reasons include:

(1) a decline in fecundity and its range (due to an increase in the age at **menarche**);
(2) increasing rates of sterility in males and females (due to environmental and dietary factors);
(3) reduced frequency of intercourse (due to increased demands on our time); and
(4) increased personal hygiene.

Mortality and Life Expectancy

Mortality refers to deaths in the population. What is important is (1) the age at which it occurs and (2) the rate at which it occurs. The rate of mortality can be calculated by gender, ethnicity, occupation and class. The general health of a nation is usually reflected by the rate of infant mortality.

Life expectancy is the total number of years a person is expected to live. It can be calculated from the fertility and mortality rates. For example, the life expectancy for females born in Canada in 1981 was 78.94. Throughout history, gains in life expectancy have been associated with a drop in the rates of infant mortality, but recently this has been changing. The increase in life expectancy is now due to the elderly living longer, since rates of infant mortality have been stable for some time. The greatest decrease in mortality rates has been in the older age cohorts.

TABLE 3.7

LIFE EXPECTANCY AT BIRTH FOR CANADIANS, 1931-1981

Year	Life Expectancy at Birth (Male)	Life Expectancy at Birth (Female)	Gain	
			M	F
1931	60.00	62.10		
1941	62.96	66.30	2.96	4.20
1951	66.33	70.83	3.37	4.53
1961	68.35	74.17	2.02	3.34
1971	69.34	76.36	0.99	2.19
1981	71.86	78.94	2.52	2.58

SOURCE: Adapted from J. Dumas, *Current Demographic Analysis*. Ottawa: Statistics Canada, 1984. P. 83.

Table 3.7 shows that males have gained 11.86 years and females have gained 16.84 years, from 1931 to 1981. This is quite substantial. However, as Table 3.8 shows, these gains have been in the earlier years of our lives; life expectancy decreases as we get older. Also, note the differences between the gains for males and females.

TABLE 3.8

GAINS IN LIFE EXPECTANCY, 1931-1981

	1931	**1981**	**Gain**
At Birth			
Male	60.00	71.86	11.86
Female	62.10	78.94	16.84
1 Year			
Male	64.69	71.67	6.98
Female	65.71	78.61	12.90
10 Years			
Male	57.96	62.92	4.16
Female	58.72	69.82	11.10
20 Years			
Male	49.05	53.38	4.33
Female	49.76	60.04	10.28
40 Years			
Male	31.98	34.72	2.84
Female	33.02	40.68	7.66
60 Years			
Male	16.29	17.96	1.67
Female	17.15	22.80	5.56
80 Years			
Male	5.61	6.85	1.24
Female	5.92	8.76	2.48

SOURCE: Adapted from J. Dumas, *Current Demographic Analysis*. Ottawa: Statistics Canada, 1984. P. 83-86.

Life expectancy also varies between and within provinces. Wilkins (1980b, 18) states that "while great progress has been made in the reduction of regional disparities in life expectancy, western Canada and Ontario have maintained an advantage over the East."

Migration

Since the beginning of this century, Canada has accepted more immigrants than it has released. Unfortunately, there are less data on movement within the country than between countries. The census data show general movements between provinces and cities, but fail to track the movements of individual citizens.

Internal movements of people may be important for the study of health of the population, since changes in the urban/rural composition of the population may affect the health of that population, its life expectancy, and rates of specific diseases. Recently it has been suggested that suburban residents live longer than people in the city core. However, Wilkins (1980b, 18) shows that the facts of health may not coincide with popular beliefs: "Contrary to a widespread belief in the unhealthiness of large cities . . . life expectancy is clearly greatest in the largest urban areas (metropolitan areas with over 100,000 population)."

International movements are important since the country of origin of the immigrant may have specific disease patterns which will require the special attention of our medical system (Heggenhougen and Shore 1986; Anderson 1986). Emigration has an effect on the population in general, since it changes the composition of the population.

In sum, age, sex, fertility, mortality and migration are important factors in the composition of the Canadian population. A study of these factors is vital for developing a suitable health-care system. The population is not equally affected by all diseases; therefore we should concentrate on those that are most prevalent.

The Health of the Canadian Population

Every historical period has had different causes of death which, we might say, were particular to that time. As civilization has progressed we have been able to eliminate certain causes of death, such as the bubonic plague; but we have not eliminated death (Zinsser 1935). It must be accepted that everyone will die sooner or later. One problem in the study of the causes of death is that medical science does not use the category of "natural death" or dying of old age. It seems as though medicine is engaged in a quest for the elimination of death which is, of course, impossible. Doctors are now focusing on the extension of life, on the assumption that more life is desirable. More life, however, is very costly and not necessarily qualitatively better.

The major causes of death in Canada today are called diseases of civilization, lifestyle or progress. In other words, something about our society and the way we live creates the illnesses we have.

> The five leading causes of death are . . . diseases of the circulatory system, neoplasms, violence, diseases of the respiratory system and diseases of the digestive system. (Lapierre 1984, 32)

> The cause of close to 80% of the deaths currently recorded each year in Canada [1971-1981] fall into three groups: cardiovascular diseases, cancers and violent deaths (principally motor vehicle accidents). (Dumas 1984)

The term "lifestyle diseases" assumes that medicine has little ability to treat these causes of death. We must assume that medicine has eliminated all the "bad" diseases to get us to our present point in history, where only the residue of "lifestyle diseases" now remains. Then, if society is the cause, should we not concentrate on transforming the aspects of society which cause the problem?

In *Canadian Medicine: A Study in Restricted Entry*, Ronald Hamowy compares the dates of the identification of specific diseases to their first effective treatment, and illustrates that there is a gap between the identification of a cause and the first effective treatment of a disease. His findings are shown in Table 3.9.

TABLE 3.9

INFECTIOUS DISEASES: DATES OF INTRODUCTION OF SPECIFIC MEASURES OF PROPHYLAXIS OR TREATMENT

Disease	Cause Identified*	First Effective Treatment
Cholera, asiatic	1883: *Vibrio cholerae* isolated by Robert Koch	1930s: Use of intravenous therapy
Diphtheria	1883: *Corynebacterium diphtheriae* isolated by Klebs and Loeffler	1894: Anitoxin developed
Dysentery, bacillary	1898: Identification of the *Bacillus dysenteriae* (*Shigella shigae*) by Kiyoshi Shiga	1930s: Use of intravenous therapy
Influenza	1933: Discovery of type A virus by Laidlaw, Andrews, and Wilson Smith	1938: Introduction of sulfapyridine 1946: Civilian use of antibiotics
Measles (rubeola)	1954: Virus first isolated in the laboratory of John Enders	1935: Treatment by sulfonamides, with questionable results 1963: Use of attenuated vaccines
Meningitis, cerebrospinal	1887: Meningococcus identified by Anton Weichselbaum	1938: Introduction of sulfadiazine 1946: Civilian use of antibiotics
Pneumonia (bacterial)	1886: Pneumococcus identified by Albert Fraenkel	1938: Introduction of sulfapyridine 1946: Civilian use of antibiotics
Poliomyelitis	1949: Poliovirus cultivated by Enders, Robbins, and Weller	1955: Introduction of Salk vaccine
Puerperal fever	1933: Lancefield classifies streptococci by antigenic properties, including those causing puerperal fever	1935: Introduction of sulfonamides 1946: Civilian use of penicillin and other antibiotics
Rubella	1962: Isolation of rubella virus	1969: Introduction of attenuated vaccines

Scarlet fever	1924: Linked to toxin-producing streptococci by Dick and Dick	1935: Introduction of prontosil
Smallpox	1915: Isolation of the vaccinia (cowpox) virus by Noguchi	17th century: Early use of variolation 1798: Protective vaccination with cowpox
Syphilis	1905: *Treponema pallidum* identified by Schaudinn and Hoffmann	1910: Introduction of Salvarsan 1946: Civilian use of penicillin
Tetanus	1884: Discovery of *Clostridium tetani* by Arthur Nicolaier	1890: Tetanus antitoxin developed
Tuberculosis	1882: Tubercle bacillus identified by Robert Koch	1947: Introduction of streptomycin 1954: General use of BCG vaccine
Typhoid fever	1880: Discovery of *Salmonella typhi* (*Bacillus typhosus*) by Carl Eberth	1950: Treatment with chloramphenicol
Typhus fever	1916: Discovery of *Dermacentroxenus rickettsi* by Simeon Wolbach	1950: Treatment with chloramphenicol
Whooping cough	1906: Discovery of *Haemophilus pertussis* by Bordet and Gengou	1938: Treatment with sulfonamides, with questionable effect 1952: Wide use of immunization, with variable protective effect

SOURCE: R. Hamowy, *Canadian Medicine: A Study in Restricted Entry.* Toronto: The Fraser Institute, 1984. P. 278-79.

*Earliest significant date, in cases of diseases having multiple causes.

It seems clear that modern medical practice is only part of the process of eliminating disease in society. Close to 80% of the deaths recorded each year fall into three general groups: (1) cardiovascular diseases, (2) cancer and (3) violent deaths. There is substantial medical evidence that the causes of these diseases are environmental or connected with lifestyle.

Cardiovascular Disease

For both males and females, **cardiovascular** diseases are the leading cause of death today: they account for 44.7% of male deaths and 48.8% of female deaths. These rates, however, have been improving in the past decade. Mortality rates from cardiovascular diseases have declined substantially between 1971 and 1981 for both sexes and for age groups over 35. "Most of the decreases exceed 20% and some were well over 30%" (Dumas 1984, 85).

There are two types of cardiovascular disease: **ischemic** heart disease (IHD), and **cerebrovascular** disease (CD).

Ischemic Heart Disease

Ischemic heart disease has the highest rates of cardiovascular death: 66.5% of male and 54.9% of female deaths. The major cause in this category is heart attacks, which account for 19% of all male deaths and 14.5% of all female deaths. The data gathered on deaths from IHD show that fewer Canadian women die from this cause, and also that women in this category are older than men.

Cerebrovascular Disease

This category of cardiovascular diseases is the second greatest cause of death, after IHD. Those affected are the elderly and, again, males are affected to a greater extent than females.

Cancer

The mortality rates for cancer are highest for those over 50, and are increasing for the elderly. There are different rates of cancer for males and females and each group is affected by different types of cancers. Mortality rates from lung cancer are growing rapidly, and this will probably be the greatest killer among the cancers by the end of the century (Dumas 1984, 88).

Violent Deaths

In the category of violent deaths there are two major causes: motor vehicle accidents and suicides. Both may be preventable, without medical intervention.

Motor Vehicle Accidents

Ever since the introduction of the car as a means of private transportation, car accidents have been a cause of death. Over the past 15 years these accidents have been attributable, in some way, to the lack of controls on drivers and car manufacturers. There are different rates by age (the 15-25 age group being the worst) and by gender. In 1982, the mortality rate for men was 24 per 100,000 and for women 9 per 100,000. Figure 3.2 shows accidents by type and sex.

FIGURE 3.2

ACCIDENTS BY TYPE AND SEX, 1969-1980

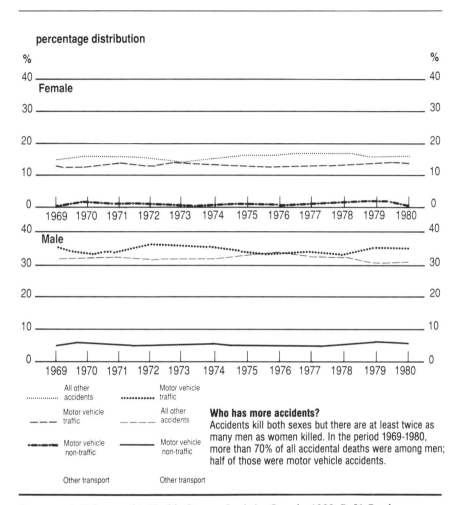

Who has more accidents?
Accidents kill both sexes but there are at least twice as many men as women killed. In the period 1969-1980, more than 70% of all accidental deaths were among men; half of those were motor vehicle accidents.

SOURCE: *In Sickness and in Health.* Ottawa: Statistics Canada, 1983. P. 21 Catalogue 82-541. Reproduced with permission of the Minister of Supply and Services Canada.

Suicides

Even though suicide is not a major cause of death in Canada it may be an index for certain social problems, as Durkheim has pointed out in his book, *Suicide.* Suicides have been on the rise in Canada since the 1950s, especially among the young. In 1982 there were 3,523 suicides. There were three times as many males as females, but there was little variation by age.

Epidemiology

Epidemiology, as stated above, is the study of the distribution and determinants of diseases within a specific population. The questions to be asked are: who gets ill, why do they get ill, and how should they be treated? To answer these questions, the patterns of mortality and morbidity in the population must first be analyzed. Next, the etiology of the disease must be considered, and there can be much controversy over this. The last item is what happens to a person after he or she has an illness. The general purpose of epidemiology is not to find the single cause of a disease, but to stop the spread of the disease.

The most famous epidemiological study was the one done by John Snow on cholera in 19th-century London. Snow looked for patterns that were common to all the victims, and by sifting through the material he found the "culprit" to be water from the Broad Street pump. (At the time there was no notion of germs or the ways in which diseases are spread.)

> In studying the 1848 London cholera epidemic he [Snow] found that people who had drunk water provided by a particular water company were much more likely to contract the disease than those who had not. The company in question drew its water from the Thames near a point where vast quantities of sewage were discharged. This supported the hypothesis that the disease was transmitted by something carried in drinking water as opposed to hypotheses involving direct transmission between individuals, which were current at the time. (Ross et al. 1985b, 33)

It is very difficult for the epidemiologist, like the sociologist, to study the whole population. Often researchers must take only a sample of the population and work on that sample. Therefore, a knowledge of sampling techniques and research methodology is a necessary prerequisite for epidemiologic studies (Rose and Barker 1979, 2). It is crucial to focus on the high-risk groups in the population, and many problems and erroneous conclusions can arise from the incorrect choice of a risk group.

Many of the methods used in epidemiology are similar to those of demography, since both look at numerical changes in a population or community. The following section will first explain some of the basic concepts used in epidemiological studies and then compare the two approaches within the field. As in demography, "epidemiological evidence about causation is often circumstantial and incomplete" (Rose and Barker 1979, 39). Both demography and epidemiology are better thought of as guides to action rather than as answers to questions.

Measuring Disease

In looking at a disease as it affects a particular population, two different rates must be calculated: the *incidence rate* and the *prevalence rate*. These rates allow us to compare different groups in the population to see if any particular group has higher rates of mortality or morbidity than the others. If this is the case, the researcher will then ask what is it about this particular group which gives it a particularly high or low rate of the illness. The incidence rate is the number of people who begin to contract a disease within a given period of time. The prevalence rate is the number of those who have the disease within a given time period.

The formula for calculating the incidence rate is

$$\frac{\text{number of new cases over a period}}{\text{population at risk}}$$

Note that people *already* ill must not be included in either the population at risk (the denominator) or in the number of new cases (the numerator). Another consideration is that an illness may occur more than once in the same individual; usually the incidence rate counts only the first occurrence of the illness.

The formula for calculating the prevalence rate is

$$\frac{\text{total number of cases at a certain time}}{\text{population at risk}}$$

Prevalence rates are appropriate only for stable or chronic conditions. They are not suitable for acute illnesses, which have a very short duration.

> Even in a chronic disease the manifestations are often intermittent. In consequence, a "point" prevalence rate, based on a single examination at one point in time, tends to underestimate the condition's total frequency. If repeated assessments of the same individuals are possible, a better measure is the *period prevalence* rate, defined as *the proportion of a defined group having a condition at any time within a stated period*. (Rose and Barker 1979, 8)

There is a relation between incidence and prevalence. The new case, or incidence, of the illness enters the prevalence pool and remains there until the individual dies or recovers. If mortality and recovery rates are low then the chronicity of the illness is high, since prevalence is equal to incidence multiplied by the average duration of the illness.

Two Approaches to Epidemiology

There is a link between the incidence and prevalence of disease in a community and the physiological and environmental status of that community. Epidemiology, therefore, must take account of the relations between people, their diseases and their environment. The process of illness must be understood in order to know the stages at which intervention is possible. The level of medical and social intervention will also vary with the type of disease or illness.

Certain assumptions are implicit in epidemiology: we want to prevent, if possible, disease from happening, stop it once it has occurred, and
help in the patients' recovery. Medical intervention can occur at three
different states. *Primary* intervention concentrates on the general health
of the population and attempts to recommend measures that can be used
before a disease arises.[5] *Secondary* intervention occurs at the stage of early
detection of a disease, the stage at which medicine can, theoretically, have
its greatest impact.[6] Lastly, *tertiary* intervention takes place at the stage of
rehabilitation or disability, with the aim of assisting resolution and
recovery.

As the above suggests, important factors in epidemiology are: (1)
what people do, (2) where they live, and (3) who they are in the society.
The causal factors would include:

(1) the biological (bacteria, viruses, insects);
(2) the nutritional (type of diet);
(3) the chemical (pollutants in the atmosphere);
(4) the physical (the climate, vegetation);
(5) the social (class, gender, occupation, place of residence).

We can assume that the distribution of diseases varies by society, and
that particular diseases are associated with certain social categories.
There are two possible approaches to the study of the effects of these
factors on the population. These approaches are (1) the traditional and
(2) the materialist. These two approaches use similar methods but are
different in their focus and prescription for health.

The Traditional Approach

The traditional epidemiological approach focuses on individuals.[7]
That is, explanations for diseases or illnesses are based on people's
lifestyle. Included are:

(1) personal habits (diet, exercise, drinking);
(2) stress/pressure (individual responses to the environment);
(3) moral traits (faults in character).

This approach suggests that individuals alter their lifestyle in order
to decrease the risk of getting a particular disease.[8] The assumption is
that the environment (social, economic, political and natural) is neutral
and does not cause or affect ill health, that is, the origins of the problem
are within the individual. Each individual is seen as having a number of
choices; if the wrong choice is made, it is the individual who is at fault.
Prevention, then, in this perspective, is defined as an individual responsibility.

The model used by this approach is *linear*. Cause is seen as an independent entity (e.g. smoking) which leads to the development of a specific disease (e.g. cancer).

$$X \longrightarrow A$$

(smoking) $\longrightarrow$ (cancer)

This model is one-dimensional and does not consider the fact that an individual's general well-being might prevent illness (Mausner and Kramer 1985, 24-39). Cause and effect, viewed from this perspective, are discrete entities, each separate from the other. This approach assumes that if we eliminate smoking, then cancer will disappear. Several criticisms can be made: a particular life situation, such as unemployment, might lead to different outcomes and indirectly to a set of symptoms.

But of course the sequence does not stop with lung cancer. There are also the consequences or outcomes of the disease. Thus:

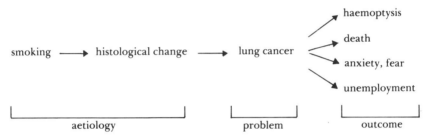

These outcomes will vary in type – some biological, some psychological, some social – and they will vary over time. . . . The diagram should take account of the fact that –

i. Smoking itself is part of a longer causal sequence:

e.g. stress $\longrightarrow$ smoking.

ii. Smoking is a part of other causal sequences:

e.g. smoking $\longrightarrow$ chronic bronchitis.

iii. The cause of lung cancer is undoubtedly multifactorial:

e.g. smoking

genetic predisposition $\longrightarrow$ lung cancer

(Armstrong 1983, 90-1)

A variation of the traditional approach, which has gained support, sees the individual within his or her lifestyle. However, there is a larger social environment which may be difficult to perceive or to control.

We can think of examples that lend validity to the above argument, such as the relation between health and diet. There is strong evidence, obtained through comparative analysis, that the way we eat may contribute to our health or illness. Estimates are that 30% to 40% of deaths from cancer could be prevented by better diet. A lack of dietary fibre, for one thing, could be the cause of a number of different diseases (Rose and Barker 1979, 38). Also, cross-cultural data show that nations, such as Japan, which have low levels of **cholesterol** consumption have significantly lower levels of heart disease than those, like Canada, that have high levels of cholesterol consumption.

We could deduce from this that the rates of certain diseases could be reduced if only people would eat the right foods. And this would not be wrong. However, most researchers now ask questions which go further. For example, are individuals *able* to change their diet, or their lifestyles in general, in order to improve their health? Does everyone have access to better food, and to knowledge about diet and health? How easy is it to purchase healthy food? Are food manufacturers committed to healthy food and ingredients? These questions have caused many epidemiologists to become dissatisfied with the traditional approach, and to move to the materialist approach.

The Materialist Approach

This approach emphasizes the larger issues of society, economy and polity to explain the patterns of disease which exist today.[9] The environment (physical and social) is not seen as neutral, but as an active participant in the health of the population. It forms the context in which we live, eat and breathe and the context within which disease arises and medicine is practised (Doyal 1983).

Researchers tell us that certain diseases arise in a particular historical context (Zinsser 1935). For example, since the 1920s there has been 20- to 30-fold rise in the number of patients suffering from **coronary heart disease**. Yet in the late 19th century the famous Canadian clinician, Dr. William Osler, was not aware of any condition involving chest pain leading to heart disease. He saw no predominant clinical pattern which would lead him to think that this condition was a major concern. J.B. Herrick was the first to document coronary heart disease in 1912. Why has there been this tremendous increase since the 1920s? What has transpired in our environment to give rise to this phenomenon? Does the explanation lie in (1) the transformation of the way individuals relate to each other, (2) the changes in industrial production, or (3) the development of cigarettes in the 1890s? Or is it a combination of all these?

Particular diseases can be linked not only with environment (for example rates of lung cancer are 30% higher in Hamilton and Windsor than in Ottawa and London), but also with the type of work done, as in the relation between mining and lung cancer. There is ample evidence that living or working in a particular environment leads to a greater risk of contracting or even dying of a certain disease. In many cases it is beyond the individual's power to control or remedy the situation. Often a choice must be made between two unhealthy situations, such as either working in a hazardous setting or being unemployed. The former at least allows the workers to feed their families. Materialist epidemiologists go as far as to say that the types of illness we are experiencing today are a product of an industrial capitalist society. Stress, which seems to be the precipitant of many illnesses, is so embedded in our way of life that we now consider it normal or even beneficial.

The model proposed by the materialist approach is complex since it sees interrelationships among (1) our social relationships, (2) our type of society, (3) factors that predispose us to disease, (4) biological changes in individuals, and (5) categories of disease. Although we separate these factors to analyze them, we must remember that they are interrelated.

Case Study

In a paper presented in 1980, Russell Wilkins analyzed Montreal mortality rates from 1961 to 1976. He found that in Montreal there was a close relationship between social class and health, by district. "It was found that the hierarchy of districts by life expectancy, mortality and survivorship correlates exceptionally well with the hierarchy of these areas in terms of income, education and occupation" (Wilkins 1980a, 2). (See Table 3.10.)

In his study Wilkins first divided the city into five zones, which he found to be segregated according to social class. Zone 1 was the wealthy area (Westmount, Outremont and Mount Royal), while zone 5 (Little Burgundy and St. Jacques) was the poor area where the welfare-dependent population lived. For each zone he looked at language, income, occupation, education, single-parent families, households without cars, and unemployment. To these he related life expectancy, infant mortality, and age-specific mortality rates.

Thus, by using techniques of population analysis, Wilkins was able to see the relation between social class and health. Some researchers may argue that further work needs to be done on the Montreal environment with respect to industry, pollution, congestion, traffic and possible other health hazards. This further research might be able to show the relationship between social classes and living conditions. It might also look at the possibility of wealthy families living in poor areas (as when older areas of the city are taken over by urban professionals) and poor families living in wealthy areas (as in the case of servants).

TABLE 3.10

SOCIAL DISPARITIES IN LIFE EXPECTANCY BY DISTRICT, MONTREAL, 1976

District	Life Expectancy	Percentage of Population
Notre-Dame-de-Grâce	75.6	6.9
Côte-des-Neiges	75.4	8.8
Ahuntsic	73.4	11.8
Saint-Michel	73.4	8.0
Villeray	72.7	12.6
Rosemont	72.1	10.0
Mercier	71.1	8.8
Plateau Mont-Royal	70.8	11.6
Sud-Ouest	69.7	7.3
Centre	68.4	8.4
Sud-Est	68.2	5.9
Montreal	71.9	100.0

SOURCE: R. Wilkins, *Health Status in Canada, 1926-1976*. Occasional Paper No. 13. Montreal: Institute for Research on Public Policy, 1980. P. 36.

NOTE: Averages of life expectancies calculated separately for each sex. Rivière-des-Prairies area excluded because of small population.

Summary

The main points of this chapter are: (1) demography and epidemiology are the basis of population medicine; (2) different populations can have specific types of illnesses which in turn influence the demands for certain types of health care; (3) the composition of the population depends on the factors of age, sex, fertility, mortality and migration; (4) the main causes of death in the Canadian population are cardiovascular disease, cancer and violent deaths; (5) disease can be measured by its incidence and prevalence; and (6) the two approaches to epidemiology are the traditional and the materialist. This chapter is a brief introduction to the methods of demography and epidemiology. There are many sources to consult if you wish to pursue these studies.

Notes

1. The *natural increase* for a specific area is obtained by subtracting the number of deaths from the number of births.
2. Rates indicate how many people, out of a population of 1,000, have a specific condition. For example, in 1983 the estimated crude death rate in Canada was 7.0; this means that for every 1,000 persons in Canada in 1983, 7 died. Percentages, on the other hand, indicate the number of cases per hundred.
3. Population aging, although caused by a number of factors, is due in large part to a declining fertility rate. Immigration is also an important factor affecting population aging in Canada.
4. Large amounts of money are available for research on certain diseases, and certain ailments are supported by our health-care system. Not all diseases are supported equally, and there are neither facilities nor programs for every illness. Funding decisions may be made on utilitarian principles, for the greatest good, or for particular political or ideological reasons. In addition, there is always more money available for primary research than for education and preventive medicine.
5. It is interesting that many physicians will not use the logic of primary prevention to focus on and eliminate hazards in the environment, but they will surgically remove parts of the body simply because they may become subject to disease. For example, many physicians recommend hysterectomies (removal of the uterus) for women past their child-bearing years (and in Manitoba, for women over 40, the ovaries are routinely removed along with the uterus). Radical mastectomies (breast removal) also fall within this category of "prevention."
6. For certain diseases, such as some cancers, early detection is no prevention at all.
7. Evidence of the popularity of this approach can be seen in the Lalonde report.
8. The logic here is that if you refuse to travel in a car you reduce the probability of getting injured in a car accident.
9. This approach does not have much support since it calls for major transformations in the society.

Chapter 4

Inequalities in Health and Illness

Health and disease are not equally distributed in society. Some Canadians, by virtue of their gender, social class or ethnic group, have a greater chance of being ill or dying early. In other words, our health and access to health care is influenced by our social situation and the activities in which we are engaged. For example, even though life expectancy for native Canadians is far below that of the national average, there is no reason to believe that this has always been or always will be the case. The rates of mortality can change for native Canadians just as for any other group. (Social inferiority should not be blamed on biological inferiority, which is a myth.)

This chapter will stress that some social groups have higher rates of mortality and morbidity, not because of their genetic or biological make-up, but because of their social position. It is true that some of us have "evident and pervasive limitations" (Gould 1985, 197), as do the mentally retarded, but even so, all people should be treated as full human beings in all respects.[1]

Before going on to analyze health inequalities by gender, social class and ethnicity, the following section will discuss (1) the difference between category and structure in health, and (2) the natural basis of equality.

Category and Structure in Health

Categories are concepts used to organize material for study. Categories are defined by researchers to enable them to divide the population into groups, according to social characteristics; this is also called taxonomy. Grouping people by the category of gender, for example, can enable us to see the differences and similarities between males and females in relation to health, illness and use of the health-care system. We can compare rates of health; for example, females have a greater life expectancy than males. Once the population is divided into different categories we can look for reasons why one category is different from another. The differences in health, however, are not biologically determined, for the most part. It may be erroneous to say that there is something about females that makes them live longer than males. Granted, females are biologically different from males, but the difference may not be as great as we think (Sevely 1987).

Gender roles are socially defined and only in certain societies do women live longer than men (Waldron 1986). If life expectancy were determined biologically, then the type of society should have little effect on differences in life expectancy. Unfortunately for sociology, there is no society where social factors are neutral or where women and men are treated the same. To understand the differences or changes between categories such as female and male, we need them to look at the structure of Canadian society.

Coulson and Riddell (1980, 33) define structure as a relationship between the individual and the society in which he or she lives. To understand the patterns of social behaviour (e.g. mortality) specific to a society, researchers must look at the society as a whole. The structure of a society affects that society's patterns of health and health care. The focus of this chapter is the way in which Canadian social structure patterns health and illness within different social categories.

> The way a society is organized might be thought of as affecting an individual's behaviour directly, by compelling people to do something, or by stopping them from doing something. (Coulson and Riddell 1980, 40-41)

Canada is an industrial capitalist society. This type of society has certain consequences for the patterns of health and illness. Industrialization itself affects the types of diseases we have (cancer for example), but also affects the types of health patterns we have (low infant mortality for example). Within capitalism, ". . . it is ultimately profit, rather than a concern to improve overall living standards, which is the most important determinant of economic and social decision-making . . . this will be reflected in various ways in patterns of health and illness" (Doyal 1979, 23).

The profit motive is the basis of all institutions within a market economy. This includes health care, once we start to label it as a commodity to be bought and sold. Although part of the health-care system in Canada is state controlled (e.g. hospitals), there is growing pressure to bring in private enterprise to run health-care services (clinics, hospitals, laboratories and chronic care facilities) because it is thought that private enterprise would be more efficient and save taxpayers' money. However, there is no evidence to support this claim and the notion of providing health for gain goes against the general thrust of Canadian history and values. In the case of Britain, the destruction of the National Health Service is based more on political philosophy than sound economic thinking. The development of private medicine in that country is creating a two-tier system, one for the rich and one for the poor (Hart 1985, Chapter 3; Turner 1987, Chapter 9).

Competition is thought to be good in our society: it makes people work harder and in theory brings the best people to the top. But what happens to those who do not "make it" and who are physically and mentally destroyed by this system? It must be recognized that our way of life produces casualties. Recent studies on the relation between stress and illness have found that all members of the society are subject to stress, not only businessmen (Beavis 1988).

Both category and structure are important to an understanding of health and illness in Canada.

The Natural Basis of Equality

Social inequalities such as those of gender, social class and ethnicity are reinforced by the common belief that the social differences which position humans in a hierarchy of wealth, power and health reflect the hierarchy in nature (Haralambos 1980, 27). That is, many people assume that inequality in social organization is based on a "natural" inequality. (It is curious that "natural" or "nature" is seldom defined in this connection).

This assumption has been backed up recently by orthodox sociobiologists, who have said that the inequalities in genetic structure determine social inequalities, and there is little we can do about social inequality. They argue that humans are part of nature, and that since nature has inequalities, so must human society. On the other hand, many sociologists, following Jean-Jacques Rousseau, "... believe that biologically based inequalities between men [are] small and relatively unimportant whereas socially created inequalities provide the major basis for systems of social stratification" (in Haralambos 1980, 27). This difference of opinion seems to leave us with an either/or choice: either society determines or causes certain patterns of inequality, or biology determines or causes them. However, the truth is probably less simple than this rigid dichotomy would indicate. We must attempt to perceive inequality in a different way, a way that does not separate the biological from the social.

Stephen J. Gould (1985, 185-98) proposes another way of looking at inequality. He sees humans as linked with nature, but he does not see nature as having inequalities. Instead, Gould says that nature has *variations*. These variations have been shaped into hierarchies by human society, which imposes a moral order on nature. That is, nature is neutral and the definitions of better/worse, good/bad and able/unable are socially derived. Biology creates differences, and society ranks these differences into a hierarchy. For example, male and female are biological differences, but society creates the inequalities by defining males as more valuable to society.

Our biology or genetic inheritance does not create the roles governing human interactions (Gould 1985, 186) and social inequalities cannot be likened to biological or genetic differences. Therefore, interactions or inequalities seen among various animals groups cannot be used as justifications for social inequalities. It is interesting that when people want to make a point about how inequalities in human society should follow those of other animal groups (e.g. the male as dominant) they pick examples that will support their case, while ignoring the many other examples that would refute it.

In the following sections on gender, class and ethnicity it is important to keep in mind the general principles of the difference between category and structure, and the understanding that social inequalities cannot be blamed on biological variation.

Gender

Since the 1970s much has been written about the discrimination against women in Canada (Armstrong and Armstrong 1983). This literature on the social situation of women has given rise to an increasing amount of research on the health of women and on sex discrimination within the health-care system (Weaver and Garrett 1978; Levinson 1976; and Bullough and Bullough 1975). Further, this literature shows that the ideas and practices of the medical system are neither neutral nor objective when dealing with women's issues or problems (Davis 1984) and that women's health patterns are influenced by their social roles. In fact, women's problems, especially those associated with reproductive ability, tend to be put into a special category and treated as unique. Rarely do we hear any reference to "men's problems" or "male syndromes."

Recent work shows that medical practice and ideology perpetuate the myth of female frailty (Suleiman 1986). This myth tends to support various medical explanations for female behaviour (Showalter 1985). Typically it is thought that a woman's inability to cope with personal or social problems is rooted in some biological flaw, as in the case of the premenstrual syndrome (PMS), which is a *normal* experience. Labelling this natural condition as a "syndrome" makes it something to be remedied by the medical profession. In reaction to this medicalization of "female problems," many women's groups have advocated the demystification of medical practice and knowledge, and the development of grassroots, self-help networks (Doyal 1983). The publication of *Our Bodies, Ourselves* (the first edition appeared in 1973) and the development of Canadian women's magazines such as *Healthsharing* are part of a developing women's health movement. This movement, in attempting to lessen medicine's control, has led to an interest in holistic medicine not only by women's groups but by all groups concerned with better health.

For example, women in Manitoba have organized a group called "Women's Health Interaction." The group's goals are:

> (1) to promote a health care system which is informed, responsible, and respectful of women's needs; (2) to demystify medical knowledge by increasing women's self knowledge; (3) to change the dependent "doctor-patient" relationship, so that health-care personnel become more like health facilitators; (4) to lobby and advocate on issues affecting women's health; (5) to empower women to participate actively in their care, and expect to be consulted and informed; (6) to link with other provincial, national, and international networks; (7) to educate individual women and providers of health care about issues pertaining to women's health; (8) to be a resource for information on any/all aspects of health care; and (9) to promote continuation of a health-care system that is universal and accessible, and to ensure that provision of health-care services be dependent upon need rather than profit. (Women's Health Interaction of Manitoba, 1986)

A basic assumption of critical, medical sociology is that our health-care system is part of the Canadian social structure, and not separate from it (Coburn et al. 1987). Therefore, the discriminatory social relationships and ideas about female inferiority which prevail in Canadian society are also embedded within the health-care system (Fidell 1980). Many even say that the medical system, because of its conservative tradition, has a greater degree of sexism and paternalism than other sectors of Canadian society. The constant focusing on women as different from men and in need of special attention has led the medical profession to focus on women's problems as the ones to be corrected. It must be acknowledged, however, that the health-care system and its methods of conceptualizing and speaking of women's problems developed historically in a context of male domination (Borges 1986). Mumford (1983, 280) says that most doctors in the late nineteenth century "... had little understanding of female physiology and anatomy, a situation which should have called for caution, but which in fact left many physicians free to invent their own theories." Unfortunately, these Victorian ideas have clouded much thinking on women's health (Bassuk 1986).

Women's health issues have only recently become a legitimate area of sociological research. Women's clinics and women's health-care groups have recently been established. There is no guarantee that these clinics will treat women differently from "mainstream" medicine, but on the whole it is probable that the development of separate women's clinics is a positive step in the progression of treatment for the whole Canadian population. There is little indication that change will come from male physicians. Fidell (1980, 327) recommends the following steps for the elimination of sexism in health care:

a) bolstering the historical and social science components of regular medical education; b) reducing sexism during medical training, in lectures, in textbooks, and in journals; c) minimizing power differences between physicians and patients to promote better communication; d) providing referral and alternative treatment facilities for the economic, sexual, political, and social problems that are inappropriately taken to physicians; e) promoting the widest possible education concerning health and treatment so that patients can intelligently select among physicians and among treatment strategies; and f) collecting solid empirical evidence concerning the efficacy of various practices and treatments.

The contribution of the women's health movement has been great because it reveals people's potential, both as individuals and as groups, to control their own lives, in spite of technology and science. Because of its fight against traditional medical practice, the women's movement is at the forefront of change in our present system of health care. Many women's groups argue that this critique must be ongoing and must include all areas in which what is male has been defined as normal and what is female has been defined as abnormal. This argument in fact is not limited to health care but extends to all "aspects of contemporary society that make women sick" (Doyal 1983, 21).

Hillier (1982b, 149) points to four reasons for studying women's health issues separately: (1) there are different disease patterns for males and females; (2) the definitions of female illness are good examples of the intrusion of social definitions into scientific medicine; (3) male and female patients are subject to the gender stereotypes which exist in the larger society; and (4) women form a majority of the labour force in the health-care system but do not occupy positions of power. These points will be illustrated for the Canadian case.

Patterns of Health

The different health patterns for males and females in Canada contradict the myth of male superiority. For each marital status category (single, married, widowed and divorced) women live longer than men. In the category of life expectancy in good health, which takes into account disability years, women also live longer than men. This was not the situation in earlier times. Before the recent reduction in family size and advances in birthing practices, many women died during child-bearing (Hollingsworth 1969, 180, 290 and 376). Women's life expectancy grew with the reduction in family size and maternal mortality. On the other hand, as women have entered the labour force and participated in stressful work relations, they have begun to show the same patterns of morbidity as men have. Previously it had been thought that men had higher rates of heart attacks because of their gender; now this susceptibility is seen to be related to work situation rather than gender (England 1988).

In Canada today women not only live longer than men, they also have a better chance of surviving at birth. Infant mortality rates for 1971-1972 were 19.5 for males and 15.1 for females. In fact, in every age group, mortality is higher for males. General cancer rates, too, are higher for males than for females (Peron and Strohmenger 1985). It is ironic that our society generally believes in male superiority, while the evidence on the ability to biologically survive supports women. One explanation for the myth of male superiority may be that our society values certain types of strength, such as physical and upper body strength, and that those who have such characteristics enjoy a better social position.

There is no doubt a physiological limit to how long we can live, and this limit may be affected by the social position of our gender. Because of the complicated nature of social life, categories such as male and female are not as simple as we might wish, as Waldron (1986, 58) concludes from her study on why women live longer:

> ... contributors to men's excess mortality involve a behaviour which is more socially acceptable for males than for females, for example aggressive competitiveness, working at physically hazardous jobs, drinking alcohol and, especially in the early part of the century, smoking cigarettes. The sex differential in smoking and alcohol consumption seems also to be linked to underlying attitudes, such as rebelliousness and achievement striving.

Morbidity (sickness) rates are a different story. Women use the health-care system more than men and have higher rates of morbidity. "Women are more likely, for example, to suffer disability from strokes, rheumatoid arthritis, diabetes and varicose veins" (Hillier 1982b, 151). Morbidity increases with age and women do live longer. Nathanson (1978, 22-23) states that even when conditions associated with childbirth are excluded, women have higher rates of morbidity for: (1) reported symptoms of acute and chronic illness, (2) restricted activity and bed disability due to acute illness, and (3) physician visits and hospital discharges.

> The greater morbidity of women and their greater use of the health care system can partly be explained by the likelihood of their experiencing disabling conditions or pregnancy which necessitate the use of general practitioner or hospital services. It has also been suggested that they might report more illness than men and that their relatively high consultation rate is a function of "illness behaviour" rather than of true morbidity. (Hillier 1982b, 153)

Nathanson (1978, 25-26) points out in her review of the literature that there are three models used to explain these sex-specific morbidity rates.

> These are: 1) women *report* more illness than men because it is culturally more acceptable for them to be ill – "the ethic of health is masculine"; 2) the sick role is

relatively compatible with women's other responsibilities, and incompatible with those of men; and 3) women's assigned social roles are more stressful than those of men; consequently they *have* more illness.

Rates of morbidity are not, however, uniform among the female population. Married women report less illness than single, widowed or divorced women. Employed women report less morbidity than house-wives, and women with preschool children report less than women with older or no children (Nathanson 1978, 29).

Assumptions about Women's Health

As stated above, medical practice has incorporated many of the sexual stereotypes common in Canadian society. A typical idea is that women's reproductive role makes them weak and frail. Some old myths have been laid to rest, such as the myth of "hysteria", supposedly caused by the wandering of the womb throughout the body (Veith 1965), but new ones are developing, like PMS.

Ehrenreich and English (1978, 5) have demonstrated that embedded within medical practice is an undercurrent of sexual politics which tends to be used as a justification for inequality.

> Medical science has been one of the most powerful sources of sexist ideology in our culture. Justifications for sexual discrimination – in education, in jobs, in public life – must ultimately rest on the one thing that differentiates women from men: their bodies. Theories of male superiority ultimately rest on biology.

The male domination of women in medical practice is obscured by the aura of science that envelops the profession. Yet many medical practices adversely change the lives of women. For example: (1) the number of caesarean births in Canada is increasing; (2) new medical syndromes like PMS are invented to explain women's frailty; and (3) new birth control methods focus on women's bodies and not men's,[2] and these methods, which interfere with female physiology, as in the case of Depo-Provera, are extremely controversial and have many side effects (Green 1987). (Depo-Provera is an injectable drug which was first developed as a treatment for cancer. Subsequently it has been used as a method of contraception for women who are considered to be unable to use other methods of contraception, for example the mentally retarded. The effect of the injection lasts for at least three months. The drug can cause infertility, cancer, severe depression, reduced circulation and extreme weight gain or loss. It is being used in the Third World but is banned for use as a contraceptive in Canada and the United States.)

Femaleness is viewed as secondary and problematic, and therefore something to be fixed. The overall ideology of medical practice tends to define menstruation as abnormal and a problem for the functioning of women in the world. Medical science seems to want to make women more like men so that women can function properly in the male-defined world. Men do not have to take time off work for their problems (and if they do they are perceived as weak.) Some gynecologists go so far as to say if women are not using their reproductive "equipment," then it should be removed since it is not functional and may cause future problems. Yet doctors don't say that old men's testicles should be removed when they are not functional, even though the same preventive argument could be made.

Another aspect currently being exposed by women researching reproductive issues is the prejudice of the medical profession toward women over 35 who are first-time mothers (Mansfield 1986). The view of older women as being less likely to have a normal birth goes as far back as the 17th century, and has yet to be seriously challenged.

> The older first-time mother has been compared by one physician to a "boxer over the hill." Her muscle tone is not good enough, he says, and neither is her endurance. She knows the words but can't play the tune. Promoting this kind of prejudice are the medical textbooks, considered by some to be the most potent mechanism by which medical advice is transmitted, often uncritically; today they still state that the "elderly primigravida is somewhat more likely to encounter complications which are the result of the natural process of growing older." (Mansfield 1986, 15)

Mansfield (1986, 16) says that "medical tradition advising women to confine their childbearing to the years before age 35 has had widespread influence on the ordering of major events in their lives, on the decision to become a mother at all, on the emotional experience of pregnancy and even on the pregnancy itself."

Now that the fashion of having children early in life is changing, women are finding that the time limit on their fertility puts constraints on the rest of their lives. Women who wish to have a career, further their education or achieve other goals and also be mothers realize that they must be concerned with age. Current government policies to limit daycare and pressure women to return to their traditional family duties adds to the pressure for early childbirth. It is probably easier to start a career before having children; however, comprehensive daycare facilities are necessary in order for women to have this choice. Where daycare facilities are limited, women face the possibility that they might not be able to get their children in at all, and might have to interrupt their careers to stay home with them.

Admittedly there is a time limit on a woman's ability to have a child, but this limit is somewhere around the age of 45 to 50. So why has a boundary been set at age 35? Part of the answer must lie in the stereotyped assumptions about women in our society, the idea that pregnancy and childbirth are events fraught with danger, to be treated by medicine.

After all these years of hospital births and promotion of scientific medicine, it is hard to convince physicians and mothers that childbirth is normal and healthy and that it should be controlled by mothers rather than doctors.

There is no convincing research to show that women who are having their first child after the age of 30 should be treated as high-risk cases. Moreover, by treating these women as high risks, medicine actually adds to the risk of the mother and child, rather than reducing it.

> Since the medical community believes these women are high risk patients, they are likely to introduce a number of interventions during labour and delivery which, while believed to be necessary and intended as helpful, may actually heighten the older woman's risks. Such iatrogenic, or physician-caused, complications include the increased risk of morbidity or mortality of mother and infant from excessive reliance on cesarean section deliveries and on drugs during labour and delivery. (Mansfield 1986, 15-16)

There has been an increase in the number of caesarean sections for first-time mothers (primiparas).[3] "We know that cesarean sections are not elected for older women solely because they are experiencing labour and delivery complications, but more likely because complications are *anticipated*" (Mansfield 1986, 18). There are often side effects from the procedure, and mortality rates are higher for C-sections than for vaginal deliveries. As well, the increased use of C-sections increases the number of children born suffering from respiratory distress.[4]

It must be acknowledged that not all males, and not only males, hold these male-centred views. But as many women have stated already, the medical definition of health is linked with the experience of those who define the problem and the institutions which support their operation day in and day out. It is clear that the definitions of women and their health needs are influenced by general stereotyped assumptions of women's frailty, and also that physicians' beliefs can influence the decisions women make about their lives.

The Treatment of Patients

The different treatment of males and females within the doctor/patient relationship also reflects sexual stereotyping (Borges 1986; Davis 1984). Female patients in general, and those with "women's problems" specifically, are treated within the ideology of medical practice described above. When female patients attempt to exert their rights and point out the obvious sexism in medical practice, counter-claims of medical superiority and scientific objectivity surface to protect the physician's authority (Mumford 1983, 280).

> Members [of the medical profession] in any conversational context will be oriented to gender as a social "fact" and engage in constructing it on various levels in the course

of their talk. Thus, for example the GP will have his medical view of women and their (specific) ailments, perhaps tempered by the more modern medical ideologies. He will have his own cultural background; the everyday notions about women prevalent in his own society as well as the relative position women occupy in it; his own experiences with women in general and his women patients in particular; his idiosyncratic response to the individual women in his office, etc. (Davis 1984, 216)

Besides the obvious fact that a majority of physicians in Canada are male (almost 80% in 1981), a majority of specialists dealing specifically with "women's problems" are male, and a majority of patients are female, so that there is a continuance of the stereotyping of women's problems through education and example. Morality and sexual discrimination are incorporated into the way physicians treat their patients.

In 1979, Armitage and others studied the way physicians treated their male and female patients. The study looked at five similar types of problems to find how well the patients were treated (the content of the treatment) and how much the patients were treated (the extent). In the majority of the cases, males received more treatment and their problems were considered to be more serious (on the assumption that males see a doctor only when they have to). Females, on the other hand, were viewed as more neurotic and more prone to hypochondria.

Another example of the lack of respect accorded to female patients is the case of abortion. Today, there are inequalities in the provision of therapeutic abortions from one part of Canada to another. These inequalities cannot be explained in terms of the available facilities.

In a study of a clinic which gave antenatal care and also referred patients for abortion, different responses to the pregnancies of single and married women were noted. For the former, pregnancy was assumed to be a disaster, for the latter a "happy event" .... Single women seeking abortions tended to be labelled "bad girls", "good girls who've made a mistake" or "almost married". In the case of single pregnant women, the question of marriage was seen as crucial and doctors often felt it legitimate to obtain some understanding of the patient's "character". They posed such questions as "who is the father of your baby?" and "are you still sleeping with him?", questions which are never asked of married women. (Hillier 1982b, 158)

Judgements about the medical procedure, the abortion itself, are clouded by the moral and cultural definitions of the type of woman who would ask for an abortion. This occurs even when the law protects the right of women to obtain an abortion on demand. There is little acceptance of the rationality of the decision to simply not have a child because of the consequences the birth of the child would have for the woman.

One important means of analyzing doctors' treatment of their female patients is to look at the way doctors are taught. For example, many medical schools do not teach their students how to do internal pelvic examinations, even though the students request this practical knowledge. Female sexuality is still viewed with the reserve which permeates the teaching of sexuality in our society (Kurtz et al. 1985). It is still a taboo.[5]

Since Canadian medical schools use the same texts and curricula as medical schools in the United States, some of the studies on that literature can be used to see how physicians are taught to view women.

Howell (1978), in her content analysis of textbooks and periodicals written by pediatricians, found a "cult of children" in which the mother was blamed for everything that went wrong with her child. "Mothers are variously blamed when their children become ill: for bothering the doctor too often, for not having brought the child in early enough, for being unduly alarmed, for not having recognized signs and symptoms of 'real' illness" (Howell 1978, 204).

Scully and Bart (1978), in their historical analysis of the portrayal of women in gynecology textbooks, found that much of the discussion was based on the idea of female inferiority. "Explanations concerning the nature of the female core are also found frequently [in texts]. Thus in 1967 we learn: 'An important feature of sex desire in the man is the urge to dominate the woman and subjugate her to his will; in the woman acquiescence to the masterful takes a high place.' Again, the female is defined as a nonaggressive, submissive, inferior being whose desire it is to be possessed by the powerful male" (Scully and Bart 1978, 220). This raises the question: what is the interpretation of a male physician when dealing with a sexually active, aggressive woman, if he has learned from such textbooks?

It is no wonder that women have begun in earnest to criticize the medical profession (Turner 1987, Chapter 5). Male attitudes about normal female behaviour have had a considerable influence on the way women perceive themselves and their relation to their children and male partners. These medical attitudes are all embedded within the larger social structure, and can be changed only with larger social change. Fortunately some physicians, including many women, have begun to be aware of the errors of their profession.

> It does not make me very comfortable to admit membership in a profession in which at least some members argue that women should be forced to bear children they do not want, fail to exert any effort to provide mothers with the means and supports that they must have to care for their children, and then invent endless ways to blame mothers for their children's misfortunes. (Howell 1978, 208)

The Gender of Health-Care Workers

Women are not only the majority of patients but also the majority of health-care workers in Canada (doctors are included in this group). As an industry, the health-care system in Canada employs mostly women. In 1980 women made up 78.7% of all hospital employees in Canada

(Armstrong and Armstrong 1983, 258). In the same year, Canadian hospitals employed 12.4% of all female workers in Canada. This was the second largest sector of employment for women, after retailing. The practice of medicine in general and the sector of hospital employment in particular are clearly sex-typed (Levitt 1977). Women employees are even more predominant in the area of chronic care, which has the lowest paid jobs.

The role of nurse has a class as well as a gender aspect, and it fits the model of the working woman today.

> A nurse's primary function is patient care – perhaps the most crucial job in the provision of health care. This aspect of medical practice, however is downgraded and derogated in terms of the hospital and medical system priorities: teaching and research. Within the area of patient care, the nurse is relegated to the role of helper – dependent on the physician for orders – even though she is often more informed of the patient's overall condition than the doctor. (Levitt 1977, 396)

Within medicine there is in fact a male/female hierarchy in which the minority of men are at the top, are paid more, and have more power and authority. In 1970-1971, physicians made up 6.4% of the total health industry labour force, while nursing and related occupations made up 51.9%. The percentage of physicians and surgeons who were female in 1970-1971 was 10.5. According to the 1981 Census of Canada there were 34,285 male doctors and 7,115 female doctors practising in Canada in 1980. In other words, over 20% of doctors were female in 1981, a doubling since 1971. The percentage of females within the medical sector who were nurses in 1970-1971 was 87.7. There are other sub-professions within the health sector as well, and the majority of these are also sex-typed.

Levitt (1977, 397) stresses that if there is to be sexual equality within the health-care industry, there will have to be more male nurses and more female doctors. The sex ratio within the medical profession may change in the future: as just noted, the percentage of female doctors doubled between 1971 and 1981. More women are being admitted to medical schools. "From 1960 to 1978, the proportion of women medical students had climbed from 9.4% to 33.3%." However, in nursing schools women are still the majority. Can we expect that with more women becoming physicians, the attitudes and focus of the profession will change? First, the increasing number of women in medicine does not mean that women will gain control of the medical hierarchy. Second, the process of selection and socialization in medical schools may in fact filter out women who do not go along with the attitudes of the current medical profession. However, people don't stop learning when they leave school: (1) women who are doctors may be influenced by social trends just as other women are, and may become more aware of the discriminatory treatment of women; and (2) women doctors may attract female patients away from male doctors, and this may force male doctors to take women more seriously.

The increase in the number of female physicians may be related to the relative incomes of doctors and nurses. Males stay out of nursing because in Canada it does not generally provide enough income to support a family. Yet many female nurses end up as the sole supporters of their families. Nurses' incomes have been relatively low for many years, even though more and more nurses have a university degree. A majority of nurses are young and work part-time to supplement the family income. Table 4.1 compares doctors' and nurses' incomes in Canada.

TABLE 4.1
INCOME OF PHYSICIANS AND SURGEONS COMPARED TO INCOME OF NURSES (REGISTERED, GRADUATE AND IN-TRAINING), 1971 and 1981 (FULL-TIME WORK)

	Physicians and Surgeons		Nurses	
	M	**F**	**M**	**F**
1971	26,990	11,054	5,795	4,566
1981	59,834	36,115	18,891	18,041

Source: *Census of Canada 1971, Income of Individuals.* Ottawa: Statistics Canada. Pp. 5-6. *Census of Canada 1981, Population: Employment Income by Occupation.* Ottawa: Statistics Canada. Pp. 5-6.

A British survey on women in medicine (Garrett 1988, 30) shows some interesting inroads women have been making in medicine. Although nearly half of newly qualified doctors are women, some specialties (e.g. surgery) attract few women, while others (e.g. family practice) attract many more. The patterns emerging are evidence of a gender division in medical careers. There may not be a conscious effort to keep women out of certain specialties, however, there is a structure which supports these divisions. For example:

> While women's careers were far more likely to have been constrained by marriage and children (and women were much more frequently asked "personal" questions in job interviews), the survey also underlined the importance of the old boy network in medicine. Men were more likely than women to have benefitted in their careers from "sponsorship" – the patronage of a senior member of the profession, who will informally put in a good word on one's behalf – and the patrons were themselves almost all men. (Garrett 1988, 30)

The position of women in the health care system is summed up by Hillier (1982b, 161): "As workers, they [women] suffer from inequality of opportunity, low status positions and poor pay, . . . [this reflects] the distribution of power and the social relationships of inferiority and superiority between men and women in society."

Social Class

There is general agreement that socioeconomic status, that is, social class or position in the economic hierarchy, determines mortality, morbidity and disability rates (Syme and Berkman 1986, 28). In Canada, income-related differences influence both the length of life and the quality of life (the latter relates to the amount of disability and unemployment) (Wilkins and Adams 1982, 26).

> Almost all the important causes of death – infant mortality, the common diseases of childhood, accidents, many cancers, chronic respiratory diseases, degenerative conditions of senescence – hit hardest at persons in the lower socioeconomic strata of society. (Last 1982, 377)

No matter how social class is defined, it is related to health and health care. This basic inequality in health exists even in those countries, such as Canada and Britain, where there is equality of access to health care and possible equality of utilization of the health-care system. It is not surprising that health and illness follow the social structural and cultural variations which are manifest in our class hierarchy. Just as gender inequalities are reflected in health and illness, so too are class inequalities (Susser, Watson and Hopper 1985, 213-275; Mechanic 1978, 163-169). Perceptions of illness, use of the health care system, and types of treatment all have class links (Fitzpatrick et al. 1984). Although there is some individual variation, a general statement can be made concerning social class and health:

> Whether the measure is overall life expectancy, disability-free life, or quality-adjusted life expectancy, the pattern is similar: the poorer you are, the less healthy you are likely to be – over a shorter lifetime. (Wilkins and Adams 1982, 25)

Illness and disease are, then, negatively correlated with social class. "English studies, for example, indicate that mortality rates in general, but especially infant and neonatal mortality rates, increase from the highest to the lowest social class" (Coe 1978, 61). Increasing mortality and morbidity rates can be seen in the entire family, not simply in the working members. In 1984, a Winnipeg study found that rates of children's illness were linked to the family income as calculated by place of residence. The city's health department began compiling data on chickenpox, lice and respiratory and gastrointestinal problems, and it found a greater prevalence of these problems in areas of the city inhabited by the poor and the working class. In British studies, higher rates of infant mortality are found in the manual labour and unskilled classes.

Recognizing the relation between social class and a particular health variable is only the start of a social explanation. The analysis must go beyond social class to the context and situation of each individual. Coe (1978, 61-62) points to three social factors which influence health: (1) environment; (2) occupation and (3) lifestyle. As Coe suggests, your health depends on who you are and the work you perform in society, not the amount of health care you receive.

Before looking at the Canadian case we need to understand how social class is operationalized (that is, put into terms that can be defined and studied) and how health data are gathered and calculated.

Health and Class

The first problem researchers have is to define "social class." There is a large amount of literature on the definition of social class, and many different ways of defining this abstract concept. Basically we know that inequality exists and that all Canadians do not have the same social **life-chances** (Hunter 1986; Clement 1983). One way of defining social class is by occupation, but there are problems with this measure; it involves developing a hierarchy of occupations. Rose and other British researchers (1985b, 78) have proposed the following criteria to develop this hierarchy, taking account of varying amounts of power, opportunity, status and mortality.

> Different occupations would differ in some of the following ways: (i) share of economic production – income, ownership of property and other durables, fringe benefits; (ii) personal control over time and activities – decision-making, rights to take a holiday or other leave, rights to allocate free time, and to choose where to work and when; (iii) mortality – health and safety at work; (iv) intellectual and personal development – education and training opportunities, scope for individual fulfillment, pleasure and enjoyment; (v) security of tenure in employment, starting date, full-time or part-time, etc; (vi) prestige – amount of social status attaching to occupation.

Another problem in defining social class is where to place the retired, children, housewives, prisoners, people who change occupations and the chronically ill. There is no doubt that the entire family is influenced by the occupation of the primary wage earner, but are all the members of the family, regardless of their occupation or lack of occupation, to be classified with the wage earner?

There is also the problem of who will collect and classify the data. This task is enormously costly in both time and money. It is difficult for any researcher to have access to and accumulate large-scale data on mortality and morbidity. If the government collects population health data in specific categories, then researchers are in many ways forced to use these data and categories. A certain amount of data is also available in non-government sociological studies.

It must be kept in mind that researchers and governments use different definitions of social class. In addition, some governments, the Canadian government for example, do not consistently keep information on the relation between health and social class. There are good administrative and political reasons for keeping statistics on the health of the population, but there are also reasons for the non-recording of mortality and morbidity. If governments fail to collect some measures of health, one explanation might be that they fear the political consequences of producing data showing that the health and longevity of Canadians is determined by their social class.

In Britain in 1911, the government department in charge of the census started using occupation as a definition of social class. The category of social class is seen in Britain as an important factor in understanding why people in certain occupations are not as healthy as those in higher paying, non-manual jobs. Table 4.2 shows some typical occupations by social class in Britain.

TABLE 4.2
TYPICAL OCCUPATIONS BY SOCIAL CLASS, BRITAIN

Social class	Examples of occupations included
I Professional, etc.	accountant, architect, chemist, company secretary, doctor, engineer, judge, lawyer, optician, scientist, solicitor, surveyor, university teacher
II Intermediate	aircraft pilot or engineer, chiropodist, farmer, laboratory assistant or technician, manager, proprietor, publican, member of parliament, nurse, pilot or fire-brigade officer, schoolteacher
III (N.) Skilled non-manual	auctioneer, cashier, clerical worker, commercial traveller, draughtsman, estate agent, sales representative, telephone supervisor secretary, shop assistant, typist,
III (M.) Skilled manual	baker, bus driver, butcher, bricklayer, carpenter, cook, electrician, hairdresser, miner (underground), policeman or fireman, railway engine driver/guard, upholsterer
IV Partly skilled	agricultural worker, barman, bus conductor, fisherman, hospital orderly, machine sewer, packer, postman, roundsman, street vendor, telephone operator
V Unskilled	charwoman, chimney sweep, kitchen hand, labourer, lorry driver's mate, office cleaner, railway porter, van guards, window cleaner

SOURCE: S. Rose et al., *Studying Health and Disease*. London: Open University Press, 1985. P. 78.

The use of this method of classification may be due to the common understanding that Britain is a class society. Table 4.3 shows the percentage of each socioeconomic group living to ages 45, 55 and 65 in 1978. (This table uses a slightly different classification than the one in Table 4.2.) From this table it is clear that the higher your socioeconomic category or social class, the longer you will live. It would seem reasonable to conclude that there is a link between the work you do and how long you will live.

TABLE 4.3

SOCIAL CLASS LIFE TABLE (MALES), BRITAIN, 1978

Socioeconomic Group	Percent Surviving from Birth		
	TO AGE 45	**TO AGE 55**	**TO AGE 65**
1. Professional	96.9	92.0	77.5
2. Managerial	96.8	91.4	76.6
3. Intermediate	96.2	89.0	72.7
4. Skilled Manual	96.1	89.3	70.7
5. Semi-Skilled Manual	95.0	87.4	69.3
6. Unskilled Manual	92.9	83.5	64.3

SOURCE: W.C. Cockerham, *Medical Sociology*. Englewood Cliffs, N.J.: Prentice-Hall, 1986. P. 51 adapted from I. Reid, *Social Class Differences in Britain*, 2nd ed. London: Basil Blackwell Ltd., 1981.

This kind of information is available because British physicians must write down on the death certificate the person's occupation, or the parent's occupation in the case of a child's death. Prior (1985) has pointed out that the data obtained from death certificates is influenced by a number of factors, including the physician's perspective on the cause of death and social pressures not to mention certain causes of death. Researchers must, then, question the objectivity of this data:

> . . . difficulties of diagnosis leave aside other significant conditions which may affect the choice of the cause of death. Thus, it is sometimes the case that certifying practitioners deliberately seek to suppress clinical data on the grounds of social sensitivity, as for example, when someone dies of alcoholism or even cancer. And other forms of social pressure may also impose themselves upon the certifying authority, as may be the case with deaths caused by asbestosis or other forms of industrial disease. (Prior 1985, 173)

Morbidity rates are higher and life expectancy rates are lower for the working class in spite of the fact that everyone is guaranteed freedom of access to the health-care system (National Health Service). Rates of use of the system do not show a vast difference between classes. But organized medicine does not prevent illness, it only treats people after they are sick, and therefore cannot halt differential rates of disease simply by providing better care or more access to care. The work that people do and their social environment have as much or more effect on their health status than does their ability to get treatment.

In the United States, the organization of health statistics by social class is less sophisticated. Illness and disease data are organized by income and not by occupation. This method of gathering and categorizing information about health originates in the ideology that the United States is a "classless" or "middle-class" society. Navarro (1977, 184-187) says this ideology stems from an assumption of homogenization of western societies, including the dissolution of the working class and its incorporation, in terms of values and consciousness, into the middle class. This process has been labelled "embourgeoisement," which means the acquiring of "an outlook and way of life that is 'middle class' " (Zeitlin 1984, 145). As a result, the category of social class has been dropped in the U.S. as an important focus of research:

> . . . analysts have concluded that past class inequalities in the distribution and consumption of resources have been superseded by persisting or newly created inequalities such as those of age, sex, [race], and regional imbalance. (Navarro 1977, 187)

The focus in the U.S. is therefore not what people do but how much they have and how much they are able to consume with what they have. Income, then, is an indicator of how much health care an individual can purchase, either from the health-care system or from the marketplace. For example, Figure 4.1 shows illness in the U.S. population in terms of income groups. Even though this gives some indication of the relation between health and social class, it assumes that the level of income is associated with the type of job.

A non-government study done in 1973 by Kitagawa and Houser (cited in Syme and Berkman 1986) on males and females aged 35 to 64 in the United States found that mortality rates varied widely by level of income, education and occupation.

> White males in the lowest educational groups have higher age-adjusted mortality rates for every cause of death for which data are available. For white females, those in the lowest educational group have an excess mortality rate for all causes except cancer of the breast and motor vehicle accidents. (In Syme and Berkman 1986, 28)

Even though the variables of education, income, occupation and "race" can be linked with health, there is no overall organizational concept of class in the U.S. which relates health to the larger occupational structure.

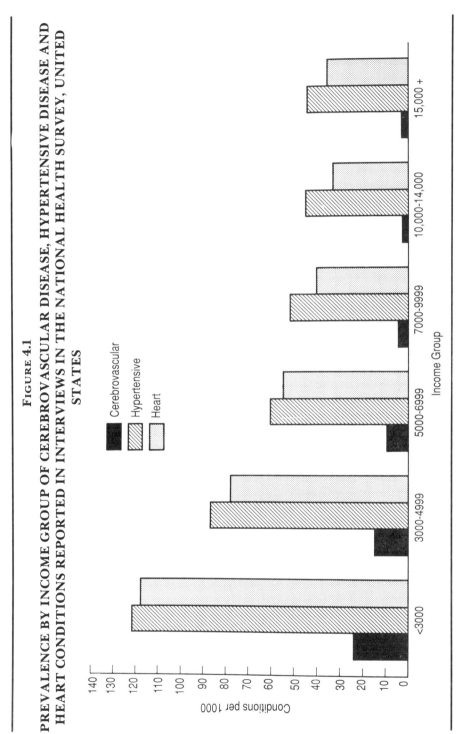

FIGURE 4.1

PREVALENCE BY INCOME GROUP OF CEREBROVASCULAR DISEASE, HYPERTENSIVE DISEASE AND HEART CONDITIONS REPORTED IN INTERVIEWS IN THE NATIONAL HEALTH SURVEY, UNITED STATES

SOURCE: M. Susser, W. Watson and K. Hopper, *Sociology in Medicine.* Oxford: Oxford University Press, 1985. P. 242 adapted from M.H. Rudov, N. Santangelo, *Health Status of Minorities and Low-Income Groups.* D.H.E.W. Publication No. (HRA) 79-627, U.S. Government Printing Office, 1979, pp. 110, 114 and 118.

In Canada too there is little information available on the relationship between social class and mortality: "Our [Canadian] mortality statistics, though they are improving in this respect, do not yet contain enough meaningful information" (Last 1982, 377). There are only a few Canadian studies that contain information on the relation between health and class. These were done on: social class in Quebec (Billette 1977), geographic areas in Montreal (Wilkins 1980a), urban areas of Canada (Wigle and Mao 1980) and occupational fatalities and illness throughout Canada (Reasons et al. 1981).

The Occupational Safety and Health Branch of Labour Canada publishes information which relates specific occupations to certain levels of illness. Table 4.4 shows how many Canadian workers were killed on the job. Although this data lends support to the argument that working-class people have a higher rate of mortality because of the work they do, government data usually underrepresent the extent of fatalities within Canadian industry. "Social Class is an important factor in one's life chances, since white-collar occupations are less risky. In a stratified, class-based society such as ours, those closer to the bottom take most of the physical risks which largely benefit those at the top" (Reasons et al. 1981, 24).

TABLE 4.4

AVERAGE FATALITY INCIDENCE RATES IN CANADIAN INDUSTRY, 1970-1978, BY OCCUPATION

Occupation	Rate per 100,000 (1970-1978)	Number of Deaths[2]	Rate per 100,000 (1978)
Mining and Quarrying	231.5	125	150
Forestry and Logging	117.0	62	100
Fishing, Hunting, Trapping	90	18	95
Transport Equipment Operation	49.2	194	35.8
Construction Trades	23.3	158	17.2
Materials Handling	19.4	48	2.3
Machining	18.3	45	5.7
Processing	16.2	63	7.9
Managerial, Administrative	8.4	54	5.7
Product Fabricating, Assembling and Repairing	6.0	54	5.1
Service	5.0	71	6.1
Other Crafts and Equipment Operating	4.8	6	5.6
Agriculture	3.8	19	1.0
Professional[1]	3.0	43	1.4
Sales	2.7	28	1.2
Clerical	1.1	19	.7

SOURCE: C. Reasons et al., *Assault on the Worker*. Toronto: Butterworths, 1981. P. 25.

1   Professional includes natural sciences, social sciences, religion, teaching, medicine, artistic and recreational.
2   This is the annual average number of deaths for the years considered.

One of the major indicators of the health of a population or specific group is mortality rates. But mortality data for Canadian social classes are not available as in Britain. For Canada, the health of social classes can be judged only by viewing specific industrial structures or by generalizing from the few studies that have been done. In a sense, researchers have to work like detectives to piece together available information to get a general sense of the health of the Canadian working population.

One of the few Canadian studies that organizes mortality data along the same lines as Britain was done on Quebec in the 1970s. Billette and Hill (1977) "examined the importance of socio-economic disparities in the mortality of working-class males. . . . If the Canadian average mortality for all males in the 15-64 age group is taken as 100, then working-age males in the lowest occupational grouping (Class V) have a relative mortality of 145, compared to a relative mortality of 75 for working-age males in the highest occupational grouping (Class I). This means that the chances of dying are nearly twice as high for males in Class V as they are for males in Class I" (Wilkins 1980a, 22). (See also Billette 1977; Beaujot and McQuillan 1982.)[6] Tables 4.5 and 4.6 show mortality levels by occupational class.

TABLE 4.5

**MORTALITY LEVEL BY OCCUPATION FOR SELECTED
CAUSES, MALES 25-64, CANADA, 1974
(AVERAGE FOR ALL CLASSES = 100)**

Cause of Death	Occupational Class*				
	I	II	III	IV	V
Lung Cancer	36	90	131	94	127
Ischemic Heart Disease	90	92	135	77	113
Cerebrovascular Diseases	87	110	90	91	117
Duodenal Ulcer	82	162	65	81	130
Stomach Cancer	66	80	80	92	172
Pneumonia	40	61	61	92	405
Bronchitis	37	55	48	68	537
Cirrhosis of the Liver	43	83	100	114	158
Accidents (non-traffic)	36	59	69	89	321

SOURCE: R. Beaujot and K. McQuillan, *Growth and Dualism.* Toronto: Gage, 1982. P. 44, excerpt from André Billette, "Les inégalités sociales de mortalité au Québec", *Recherches sociographiques,* vol. XVIII, no. 3, 1977.

Concerning morbidity, again there is little information available in relation to social class. In 1981, Statistics Canada published the findings of a health survey of 4,200 Canadians done in 1978-1979 (Canada 1981). The information collected correlated the prevalence of health problems with age, sex, activity and family income. The categories of activity used were: (1) working, (2) housekeeping, (3) school and (4) inactivity. This study reveals patterns of reporting illness and utilization of the health-care system, but little about how the type of occupation may affect morbidity (Mumford 1983, 128-129).

The measure of family income used in this survey divided the Canadian population into quintiles, each one representing 20% of the population. The first quintile was the poorest fifth of the population and the fifth quintile was the wealthiest fifth of the population. Even though this information is helpful, there are flaws in the data since the different social classes do not report illness equally. In Table 4.7, those in the fifth quintile would probably be business executives and managers and those in the first quintile, unskilled labourers or unemployed. These figures, when coupled with the mortality data above, show that rates of heart disease and mortality are highest not among executives but among skilled and unskilled workers. There are problems in using these data in comparisons with other countries, such as Britain and other European countries. For example, there is no reason why farmers are put into Class V. In Table 4.2 (the British example) farmers are put into Class II and Class III

TABLE 4.6

SOCIAL DISPARITIES IN MORTALITY AMONG MALES 25-64 BY OCCUPATIONAL CLASS, CANADA, 1974

Occupational Class	Relative Mortality	Percentage of Work Force
I Professionals and upper levels of management	75	17.7
II Technicians and middle levels of management	82	22.6
III Skilled occupations, including immediate supervisors	92	21.6
IV Semi-skilled occupations, including immediate supervisors	115	23.3
V Unskilled workers, farmers, and labourers	145	14.8
All classes	100	100.0

Note: Occupational categories according to Blishen-McRoberts Scale.

Table 4.6 – Continued

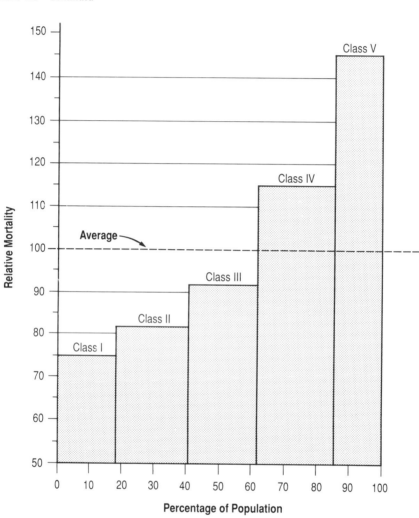

SOURCE: R. Wilkins, *Health Status in Canada, 1926-1976*. Occasional Paper No. 13.
Montreal: Institute for Research on Public Policy, 1980. P. 35 and 23.

is broken into manual and non-manual parts. Since there is no standard
way of organizing social class data from country to country these problems of comparison will continue to exist.

Also using income quintiles to measure health, Wigle and Mao
(1980) studied mortality rates in Canadian urban centres. They con-
cluded: ". . . it is clear that Canadians in lower income levels did experience substantially higher mortality rates for most diseases than persons

TABLE 4.7

PREVALENCE OF HEALTH PROBLEMS BY ECONOMIC
FAMILY INCOME, BY SELECTED HEALTH PROBLEM,
CANADA, 1978-1979

Quintile	I	II	III	IV	V
Hypertension	26.7	17.5	15.9	15.4	19.0
Heart Disease	33.0	18.3	16.0	13.9	16.0
% of quintile having one problem	20.3	18.1	17.6	18.9	20.2
% of total problems in population	23.8	18.0	17.0	17.7	19.3

SOURCE: Adapted from *The Health of Canadians.* Ottawa: Health and Welfare Canada, 1981. P. 117.

with higher incomes" (Wigle and Mao 1980, 3). "Infants of either sex and males in age groups 1 to 14 and 35 to 64 in level 5 (low income) experienced mortality rates almost twice as high as those for level 1 (high income). . . . Males in income levels 1 and 5, respectively, had life expectancies at birth of 72.5 and 66.3 years; the corresponding values for females were 77.5 and 74.6" (Wigle and Mao 1980, 1).

The general statement about class and health (that is, as social class increases, so does the standard of health) holds true in Canada. The poorest fifth of the population has a higher reported prevalence of most health problems. Improved reporting of illness or access to medical care cannot be expected to reduce deaths from environmental or social causes (Davis and Schoen 1978, 29) but may point out areas where research and health spending are needed. It is wrong to assume that major improvements to health will come from an expansion of health services or greater technology. For the working class it is obvious that improvements in health will come from a safer work environment, and that a safer environment will be one in which people, not profits, are the primary concern.

Hazards of Work

In 1978 there were over one million work injuries and illnesses among some 8.5 million Canadian workers. If we add 25 per cent to the number of injuries and illnesses to adjust for coverage of all workers in Canada, a total of about 1.33 million injuries occurred in 1978. Therefore, about 16 per cent of the workforce in Canada sustained an injury or illness on the job. (Reasons et al. 1981, 25)

We have already seen the relationship of social class to work, and of occupational level to a person's life chances.

... worker's survival depends on the "health" of the company. Workers may face the threat of plant closure or displacement by automated equipment if they press too hard for improved health and safety. And when plants close down, it is not easy for workers to go elsewhere. They transform personal circumstances and skills or break social or geographical ties at great cost to their way of life. (Sass 1980, 28)

In 1982, Allan Kalin, president of an occupational health and safety consulting firm, stated: "we spend one-third of our lives in the working environment and many of our chronic illnesses have been linked to our surroundings" (*Jager* 20 1982, 20). It is important, then, to understand and remedy the possible hazards of work if we want to solve the problem of inequalities in health.

The following statistics give an idea of the human costs: (1) every 15 minutes, 130 workers in Canada are injured on the job; (2) every year, up to 1,500 workers are killed on the job; (3) every year, 20,000 workers are permanently disabled; (4) in the next 20 years, 2 million workers will be seriously injured or die young because of industrial diseases or accidents (Sass 1980, 28).

Generally, the working class is that group which works with the most dangerous materials and in the most dangerous conditions. The health of these workers, until recently, has not been an issue of industrial development. There are many hazards which go unnoticed, or which medical experts refuse to label as dangerous (Reasons et al. 1981) or for which company doctors refuse to blame the company (Walters 1982b). It takes many years for the effects of some hazards to be noticed, so that often the cause of chronic illness cannot be traced to the company. Therefore, the courts (Brodeur 1985) and the medical profession (Sass 1980), especially company doctors (Walters 1982b), are reluctant to force industries to change their patterns of production (Reasons et al. 1981, xiv).

A recent example of the differences of opinion over the work environment is the resurgence of discussion on the safety of video display terminals (VDTs). Since 1980, newspapers have published information on the number of abnormal children born to women who work at VDTs (Chenier 1982, 26). In an article in the *Winnipeg Free Press* (Speirs 1986) the safety of VDTs was again questioned by organized labour. While cancer researchers and radiation experts have said that "radiation from VDTs poses no health threat to workers, including pregnant women," labour representatives say there is no evidence to show either that VDTs are harmless or that radiation standards are objectively established (Chenier 1982, 26).

Many health problems ... have already been associated with VDT use. ... Estimates suggest that about a quarter of a million ... video display terminal devices were in use across the country, with at least 100,000 Canadians, mainly women, spending up to eight hours a day in front of them. (Chenier 1982, 27)

If there is a possibility of harm from VDTs, should workers, especially pregnant women, be exposed to even low levels of radiation? This example points to the question that arises in almost all controversy in occupational health: *how much* (radiation, chemical exposure, etc.) *is safe?*

Other examples of workers suffering illness from conditions that turned out to be unsafe are the cases of lead-poisoning in a Winkler, Manitoba foundry (*Winnipeg Free Press*, 11 April 1986), lung-cancer deaths in the Hamilton steel industry (*The Globe and Mail*, Toronto, 30 June 1986) and miscarriages among nurses who are exposed to various gases in the Brandon Hospital surgical theatre. Other harmful features of the work environment include alienation and stress. "It's been reported that every day, approximately 350,000 workers are absent from work because of alcohol, drugs, or stress-related problems" (*Winnipeg Free Press*, 20 November 1982, 40).

Even the business cycles ("boom and bust") have an effect on mortality rates. Brenner found that "social stresses which rise with the [economic] boom are responsible for the business cycle peak of the death rate" (Eyer 1977, 625). Job pressures can be heightened during economic booms, which cause stress and higher mortality rates because of the social effects on individuals and their families. (Note that an economic boom is not more or less stressful than a depression, but each affects different groups of people differently.)

The perception of the labour movement has been that industry considers profits more valuable than lives. "It is not that management ignores the health of workers, but rather that it balances health issues against costs" (Walters 1982b, 11).

The financial costs of worker illness and injury are as follows: (1) for every day lost in Canada due to strikes and lockouts, six working days are lost through workplace accidents and disease; (2) 70 million working days were lost in 1977 because of job-related illness or injury; (3) the yearly cost of workplace accidents in Canada is over $4 billion. This staggering total includes lost wages and pensions, medical expenses, lost production, damaged machinery, administration and rehabilitation (Sass 1980, 29). These figures clearly indicate that there is little concern for the health and safety of workers (Sennett and Cobb 1972).

Moreover, there has been a tendency on the part of the courts and industry to blame the worker (Kinnersley 1973).

> By focusing upon the worker as the cause of accidents, we then look for solutions to violence in the workplace by somehow changing the worker. The victim is thus set up as the culprit, freeing the company or work environment from the blame. (Reasons et al. 1981, 137-138)

Unemployment and Health

From the above section it may appear that the work we do shortens our lives and increases the risk of getting and dying of certain diseases. Work is, however, a central human activity.

> Work has always had a profound impact on the lives of those who perform it. . . . Today adults ordinarily spend at least one-third of their waking hours on the job. What people do during these hours often penetrates to the very core of their personalities [and their health]. (Rinehart 1975, 1)

Many studies have found that being unemployed or not working is also hazardous to health (Grayson 1985). Coburn (1978, 430) suggests that ". . . various dimensions of work are indeed related to a worker's general psychological and physical well-being." Anthony and Jansen (1984, 538) state that engagement in productive work results in the rehabilitation from chronic mental illness. According to Brenner (1979, 568):

> . . . economic instability and insecurity increase the likelihood of immoderate and unsafe life habits, disruption of basic social networks, and major life stresses – in other words, the relative lack of financial and employment security of lower socioeconomic groups is a major source of their higher mortality rates.

Lack of work can be **debilitating** emotionally and even physically. In a study on the effects of plant closure, Grayson found that the health of the unemployed and their families was worse than the health of those still employed, even after a period of two years (Grayson 1985, 80).

There may seem to be a contradiction in the information presented in this section; work is both helpful and harmful to the worker. However, a distinction can be made between one's work and one's job. The job structures the work and the working environment. The way the job is organized can alienate people from their work, putting pressure on their ability to live a full life. The pressures of the job have an overall effect on an individual's life chances. The solution then is to organize work so that it does not detrimentally affect the health of the worker.

Ethnicity and Culture

The concept of "race" has entered our everyday language. Those who study health and illness, especially in the United States, commonly use the category of "race." "One reflection of social inequality in the United States is the differences among the health profiles of racial groups" (Cockerham 1986, 43). It is not clear, however, on what basis people are placed in one racial group or another. In Canada, race is not commonly used as a category in the collection of mortality and morbidity statistics[7], even though we are influenced by research and methods of data collection used in the United States.

It is illogical and fallacious to use the concept "race" to analyze social and cultural differences such as mortality and morbidity rates, since race is a biological categorization. It is a fact that the health of blacks in the United States is poorer than that of whites, and in Canada the health of natives is poorer than the health of the rest of the population. But it would be wrong to conclude that these groups are less healthy *because* they are (genetically) black or native. The biogenetic structures are basically the same for all racial groups. Physical racial traits bear no relationship to culture, behaviour or personality (Anderson and Frideres 1981, 14). Therefore, race is neither an appropriate category for the study of health and illness nor is it a good descriptive tool for showing variations in human societies. The development of a classification system based on race goes back to the beginnings of social science, and was an attempt to show the inferiority of certain non-white groups.

> We cannot understand much of the history of late nineteenth- and early twentieth-century anthropology . . . unless we appreciate its obsession with the identification and ranking of races. For many schemes of classification sought to tag the various fossils and ancestors of modern races and to use their relative age and apishness as a criterion for racial superiority. (Gould 1985, 189)

Since the category of "race" turns the focus of etiology, or cause, from the social to the biological, a better category is that of "ethnicity." Ethnicity, or culture, can be correlated with variations in health and illness in the population without the danger of hinting at racial superiority or inferiority.

Behaviour and socialization play a large part in the ways people perceive their illness, use the health system and risk getting certain diseases; therefore it is more appropriate to use categories that will help identify the social basis of these differences[8] and not concepts developed to foster an ideology of racial superiority.

Culture and Health

There is little debate over the fact that different cultural groups perceive and experience illness and disease differently (Helman 1984). The study of pain demonstrates differences between social and physiological reactions to illness. It may be hard to understand how pain can affect people differently. There are, however, two component parts of pain: (1) the sensation, and (2) the reaction to the sensation. The second ". . . includes certain changes in facial expression, grimaces, changes in demeanour or activity, as well as certain sounds made by the victim, or words used to describe his condition or appeal for help" (Helman 1984, 96). Thus, pain has social aspects, since there is a relation between the person who experiences the pain and the individuals with whom the person interacts to solicit help or sympathy.

Zola (1983, 90), summarizing the works of Margaret Mead, gives a dramatic example of the differences in the social aspects of pain:

> Arapesh women reported no pain during menstruation, quite the contrary is reported in the United States. Interestingly enough the only consistent factor related to its manifestation among American women was a learning one – those that manifested it reported having observed it in other women. . . . The fact that one has to learn that something is painful or unpleasant has been noted elsewhere.

From the above example, and other studies, it is clear that the feelings and behaviour associated with a specific medical condition are not the same for all. Yet the practice of medicine usually does not allow for these differences and tends to treat everyone in a similar way, regardless of ethnicity or culture.

Canada is a multicultural society in which different ethnic groups are allowed (at least in theory) to practise their particular culture and maintain their histories (Anderson and Frideres 1981). The survival of each cultural group depends on a number of complex factors including their institutional support (Breton 1964). There are many institutional processes in mainstream Canadian life, however, which do not take account of the different cultural pressures and demands which are put upon them. This is particularly true of medicine. The medical system tends to treat everyone, regardless of culture, as a typical "patient." The outcome is to structure the way different groups use the system or set up alternative health systems (Weidman 1981, 137). The challenge for Canada is to adapt our present medical system to the many and varied demands of the different cultural groups which make up this country. There are some signs that this is being done already.

> Across Canada native peoples are working as interpreters for doctors and nurses; the most successful program seems to be at the Children's Clinic, a Winnipeg hospital where an Indian man and four women work full-time not only as interpreters of five different dialects but also as health advocates who reassure the children, play with them, and keep their parents informed through letters and Polaroid pictures. (Grescoe 1981, 121-122)

This case, unfortunately, is not the norm, and the traditional values and beliefs of certain cultures are often viewed as "unscientific" and cumbersome to the health-care system, and even as conflicting with modern medicine (Kaufert and Koolage 1984).

> All too often . . . the cultural beliefs of patients are viewed by orthodox providers of care as irrational or superstitious, negative, and as a symptom of ignorance. They are, therefore, not taken into account in diagnosis and treatment. (Weidman 1980, 137)

If it is acknowledged that much of the process of healing is connected with the beliefs of patients, why is orthodox medicine opposed to "traditional" methods of healing? Many researchers state that the unwillingness of the medical profession to release control over the health-care system has little to do with the "scientific" basis of modern medicine, and much to do with the self-preservation of the profession (Larson 1977).

There is little health information on the different ethnic groups of Canada, either in academic articles or in government data. It is, then, almost impossible to understand the particular needs of the different cultural groups in Canada or the particular perceptions of different groups about their illnesses (Anderson 1986). However, individuals with a specific cultural heritage do not necessarily hold to the traditional beliefs. Many traditional forms of healing are not passed on to the younger generation or are illegal in Canada today. One group which has had a strong reaction to modern medicine and which is clearly adversely affected by the dominant Canadian culture is native Canadians.

The Health of Native Canadians

In 1984, there were over 300,000 treaty or status Indians in Canada, about 1.5% of the Canadian population (Young 1984, 257). It is common to think of Canadian Indians as a single homogeneous group belonging to a particular race, culture or nation. However, this is not the case. There are many different groups of natives with distinct beliefs, languages, practices and health problems. To study the patterns of health and illness among these groups would require that we treat them as separate units and collect information based on the particular characteristics of each group. Again, unfortunately, this is not done.

Most of the information kept on the health of our native peoples is lumped together in a single category – Indians. To further complicate things, the federal government distinguishes between treaty and non-treaty Indians and between Indians and Métis.

Discrimination, poverty and poor living conditions have all contributed to the poor health conditions of native Canadians. In 1977, only 11.5% of houses on reserves in Manitoba had running water.

> With cultural backgrounds widely divergent from those of the dominant Euro-Canadian society, Indians have continued to suffer from the effects of considerable political, social and economic underdevelopment. In terms of health status indicators, numerous studies and official statistics consistently demonstrate a wide gap between Indian and non-Indian Canadians. (Young 1984, 257)

The solution to this problem, if history is to be a guide, is not to force modern "white man's medicine" upon these peoples. "It has become apparent that government's efforts to improve the health of Indian people are no longer having the desired effect. Our standard medical tools do not seem to address . . . [the] accelerating crisis of health and social breakdown" (Canada 1979). Health, as has already been argued, will be enhanced by better living conditions more than by the introduction of health services. This was stated in the first stage of a new Indian Health Policy issued by the federal government in 1979. It looked to "the importance of socioeconomic, cultural and spiritual development to attack the underlying causes of ill health" (in Young 1984, 263).

Life Expectancy, Mortality and Morbidity

Life expectancy among native Canadians is significantly lower than for the rest of the population. "The average age of death for Indians, 42.4 years, is nearly 24 years younger than that of the general population" (Grescoe 1981, 110). Even though this age has increased over the past three decades, there is still a significant difference in life expectancy at birth. Table 4.8 shows native Canadians' life expectancy compared to that of the rest of the population. Life expectancy varies not only among provinces but also within the provinces, among bands.

TABLE 4.8

LIFE EXPECTANCY OF NATIVE CANADIANS, COMPARED TO NATIONAL AVERAGE
(Average Additional Years of Life)

		1961		1971	
		Male	Female	Male	Female
At 1 year	National	63.5	74.3	69.3	76.3
	Indian	59.7	63.5	60.2	66.2
At 50 years	National	24.3	28.5	24.5	29.9
	Indian	25.1	26.2	24.8	27.6
At 80 years	National	6.3	7.0	6.4	7.9
	Indian	6.0	6.6	8.0	8.9

SOURCE: *Indian Conditions: A Survey.* Ottawa: Indian and Northern Affairs Canada, 1980. P. 15. Reproduced with permission of the Minister of Supply and Services Canada.

Mortality among natives is very different from that of the rest of the Canadian population. Infant mortality rates, while declining from the rate of 79 per 1,000 in 1960, are more than twice the national average. This is also true of stillbirth rates (Bruyer 1981). The higher risk of mortality and morbidity for native infants is associated with the frequency of high and low birth weights. This is a problem which could be solved by better nutrition, monitoring, midwifery and education, but not by more medical technology. Children and young adults also have high rates of mortality, while the mortality rates for native Canadians aged 70 to 79 is lower than that of the general population (Rowe and Norris 1985; Young 1983).

The causes of death for natives are also different (Rowe and Norris 1985). There are higher mortality rates among the native population for suicides, poisonings, infections, genito-urinary and neurological diseases, and congenital anomalies (Young 1983). While native rates of cardiovascular and cancer mortality are closing on the general population rates, the largest single killers of native Canadians, especially the young, are accidents and violence.

TABLE 4.9

VIOLENT DEATHS OF NATIVES AND NON-NATIVES IN
CANADA (RATES PER 100,000)

	National (1974)	Native (1976)
Motor vehicle	26.9	60.5
Burns and fire	3.5	23.6
Firearms	0.5	21.4
Poisoning and overdose	3.0	14.9
Suicides	12.1	30.1

SOURCE: M. Best, "Indians: Victims of Failed Policy." *Winnipeg Sun*, 24 October 1982. P. 12a.

Although the rates of many diseases are higher among natives, some are lower. One example is cancer; rates of lung, breast and skin cancer are lower even though a greater proportion of natives smoke (Young and Choi 1985). Rates of cervical, kidney and gallbladder cancers are, however, higher among native populations. It has been suggested that this pattern is changing to correspond with the general population's rates, along with the environmental and cultural transformation of native peoples.

Morbidity rates among natives are also higher than those in the rest of the Canadian population. According to the Department of Indian and Northern Affairs (Canada 1980a), in 1976 the hospital admission rates for natives was higher for infectious and parasitic diseases, diseases of the nervous system, respiratory and gastrointestinal diseases, diseases related to childbirth and complications of pregnancy. General hospital admission rates for natives are more than twice the national average. Even though admission rates are high compared to the general population, we know that utilization rates (that is, use of the broader health-care system) by the native population are low due to cultural, linguistic and geographic factors. Because of the discrimination felt by native peoples, they rarely go to private physicians and will use other facilities, emergency services for example, only when necessary (Riffel et al. 1972).[9]

Alcohol and Drug Abuse

Alcohol is commonly cited as a factor contributing to the high rates of accidents and violent deaths among the native population (Jarvis and Bolt 1982). However, high rates of alcoholism among native Canadians are not caused by racial factors. The use of alcohol and drugs is related to the natives' history, social disintegration and lack of alternatives: it is a social rather than a biogenetic problem.

Within the native population, morbidity rates for drug and alcohol users are higher than for non-users. There is no information, however, to show that natives experience higher rates of mortality resulting from the chronic effects of alcohol use (Giesbrecht and Brown 1977). Another problem in native communities is glue and gas sniffing. The latter has contributed to high rates of lead poisoning and mental "slowness" (Postl 1975).

Environment

The health of native Canadians is constantly affected by changes in their physical environment. Whether it is the flooding of lands or the destruction of game, many natives are adversely affected by changes in the natural environment within which they must live in harmony. For example, many natives depend upon fish as a major part of their diet. Yet the problem of mercury-poisoned fish has become serious throughout Canada, in the English-Wabigoon River in Northern Ontario, in the Red River in Manitoba and Saskatchewan, in the Upper Howe Sound in British Columbia, and in various other fresh-water systems in Ontario, Quebec and Labrador (Canada 1980a; Sutherland 1976).

Mercury poisoning is not the only problem caused by the industrialization of the North. More and more evidence is coming to light of other problems which plague the health of natives in Canada. These problems are not the fault of the natives, but result from our society's disregard for the environment on which many natives depend. Again, the problem could be solved by prevention.

Health Services

The status of natives within Canadian society is reflected in their treatment by the health-care system. Generally speaking, the services given to natives by the health-care system are inadequate.

The federal government of Canada has been responsible for the health of treaty Indians since the enactment of the British North America Act in 1867. The famous "medicine chest" and "pestilence" clauses in Treaty No. 6 (1876), between Canada and the Crees of what are now central Alberta and Saskatchewan, initiated the responsibility of the federal government for the health of Canada's native population (Young 1984, 257-58). In 1962 this responsibility was assumed by the Department of National Health and Welfare. Since 1970, there has been a lack of active support by the federal government for treatment services for the native population. The gradual withdrawal of services was initiated in 1969 by a White Paper which suggested the provincial takeover of federal services to Indians. There was considerable reaction by the native population against this switch, since it threatened the special status of natives in Canada and the responsibility of the federal government for these peoples (Young 1984, 262).

Even though treaty Indians are guaranteed free medical service, this service has been inadequate because of the geographic consolidation of medical services in larger cities, the lack of understanding of health problems of the native population, and the natives' distrust of "white man's medicine" (Riffel et al. 1972). Health services to the scattered native population are insufficient, while the traditional health practices of native healers are being eroded by contact with modern, scientific medicine. Most of these problems, however, cannot be solved by the further introduction of medical services (Canada 1980a).

It is hard to understand why native Canadians still continue to suffer and die from diseases that were eliminated in the general Canadian population more than 30 years ago. According to Berger (1980, 4) "the problems of Indian health are the outcome of centuries of oppression, of the domination of one society by another." There is no simple solution, since health is not rooted in the services we provide but in the general living conditions of native peoples.

The higher mortality and morbidity rates among the natives in Canada have been described as a "national disgrace" (Grescoe 1981, 109), since these rates are the result of poor nutrition, inadequate housing, substandard water and sewage services, and high rates of alcohol and drug abuse. All of these factors contribute to the negative image Canadians have of native peoples, while at the same time affecting their quality of life. These problems cannot be blamed on the individual or genetic makeup of our native peoples, but are a result of their place within Canadian society.

Summary

This chapter has offered a description of the health and illness of Canadians according to three categories: social class, gender and ethnicity. The purpose was not to concentrate on the unique qualities or characteristics of these groups, or to point to biological or racial explanations for different rates of illness, but to show how the structure of society in Canada influences the health and illness of different social groups.

The main points of this chapter are: (1) in Canada today there is inequality in both health and access to health care; (2) this inequality is not based on biology; (3) the organization of our society influences the health of different social groups positively or negatively, depending on gender, class and ethnicity, (4) health and life expectancy are influenced more by what you do than who you are; and (5) cultural practices account for the types of illness people have.

Notes

1. As stated earlier, the retarded and handicapped are discriminated against because they are not able to function, and our society is organized in a way that inhibits them from doing certain functions. Yet the handicapped are able to contribute to society in productive ways, and the development of technology has assisted in their productivity.

2. Since the appearance of AIDS the Europeans have been testing a female condom. It is said to be preferable to the male condom because it feels the same for the woman but better for the man. The assumption of the researchers is that women will be more responsible for the use of the condom than men are.

3. In 1985 10% of births in Britain and 25% of births in the U.S. were C-sections. There is increasing pressure on physicians to opt for a C-section because of the possibility of being sued for the birth of a brain-damaged child (which is 1 in 3,000 to 4,000 births) (Ferriman 1988, 36). Many non-emergency C-section babies are premature since there is a desire to deliver smaller babies.

4. Again, medical intervention creates new medical problems. Jenkins (1987, 19) says that "prolonged mechanical ventilation of neonates . . . makes it difficult to wean infants from the respirator." This is because the ventilator inhibits the development of the infant's muscle fibre.

5. There have been unofficial reports of pornography being used in medical school anatomy classes.

6. In Britain the ratio between occupational classes I and V is 1:8; in France it is 1:5 (Wilkins 1980b, 22).

7. Because of new employment equity legislation, designed to improve opportunities for native and ethnic groups, Canadians may be asked to state their "race" on the 1991 census.

8. For some genetically determined diseases, such as sickle-cell anemia, race may be a factor. However, that does not mean that these racial groups are physically or socially inferior.

9. Before 1981 there were no native physicians and only 221 native nurses in Canada (Grescoe 1981, 122).

Chapter 5

The Health-Care Professions

The practice of medicine in Canada is organized around a number of specially trained occupational groups, each of which has a specific task within the medical system. By virtue of their education, training and responsibility, some groups have more power than others; there is a hierarchy of occupations within medical practice. There are 35 medical specialties, which can be ranked by income and prestige (Blishen and Carroll 1978). However, this medical hierarchy is defined not only in terms of knowledge and experience but also in terms of social class, gender and ethnicity (Shapiro 1978, Chapter 4). This chapter will consider how these groups are separated from each other and why some have more control and power than others.

All medical occupations, regardless of their position within the system, adhere to principles of medical care that are defined by physicians. That is, doctors continue to determine the manner in which health-care needs are met (Johnson 1972, 47).

The functionalist argument proposed by Davis and Moore (1945) states that society must lure its most gifted to the most important social positions. Therefore, physicians must be given high status and many incentives, so that the brightest and best will be drawn to this important work. "The greatest rewards are associated with those roles that (1) have the greatest importance for society and (2) require the greatest training of talent" (Cockerham 1986, 149). Thus, even though the practice of medicine does require certain expertise and social skills, the current high status of the medical profession within society and within the health-care system is also a product of professional power gained through political support (Conrad and Schneider 1986, 127). That is, although the work of doctoring is difficult and necessary, this work in itself does not define the social position of physicians. Their position is supported, rather, by our social value for health as well as the monopoly the medical profession has over health care. Professional power is the source of medical autonomy and dominance (Friedson 1986).

The Division of Labour in the Health-Care Professions

The tasks associated with health care have become more and more complex over the past 50 years. The **division of labour** within the health-care system has increased and created specialized groups to administer and control each task. As a result, health care is broken down into many parts. Table 5.1 shows the range of health-care occupations.

TABLE 5.1

SELECTED HEALTH OCCUPATIONS

---

(1)   Health diagnosing and treating occupations
      Physicians and surgeons
      Dentists
      Osteopaths and chiropractors
      Naturopaths and podiatrists
(2)   Nursing, therapy and related occupations
      Nursing supervisors
      Graduate nurses
      Nurses-in-training
      Nursing assistants
      Nurses' aides and orderlies
      Physiotherapists, occupational and other therapists
      Ambulance teams, first aid, home support groups
(3)   Other
      Pharmacists
      Dietitians and nutritionists
      Optometrists
      Dispensing opticians
      Radiological technologists and technicians
      Medical laboratory technologists and technicians
      Dental hygienists, assistants
(4)   Administrators

SOURCE: *Occupational Distribution of Employment: Canada and Provinces.* Ottawa: Statistics
      Canada, 1975. P. 386.

As the amount of knowledge in each medical specialty increases, so does the amount of work that must be done within that specialty, and the amount of preparation necessary to qualify for it. Since the complexity of health care is increasing rapidly and since it is almost impossible for one group to keep up with the expansion of knowledge and technology, new occupations and sub-occupations are created. At the beginning of the 20th century physicians carried out almost all of the tasks associated with health care. Since then we have seen the development of many specialty occupations which treat specific ailments or parts of the body, and of support staff to assist them. This increasing specialization has contributed to a view of the patient as a case, rather than as a whole, social person. The tasks performed in the past by doctors are now carried out by nurses, and the tasks that nurses performed are now carried out by LPNs (licensed practical nurses) and nurse's aides. However, even though the numbers of health-care specialties are increasing, physicians still maintain control over the health-care system. This is accomplished through their autonomy and their dominance over diagnosis and treatment, supported in turn by the growing division of labour. Therefore, the greater the number of specialized tasks, the less control and understanding each medical worker has.[1]

As stated previously, in our society health is seen as a commodity which is produced by a number of specialists, working as a team. The assumed goal of this team is the health of the patient. The organization of occupational groups around the principles of medical practice has traditionally increased the number of health-care workers per patient. However, this is changing because of the increased pressure to cut health-care costs, especially in hospitals and the pressure to be more efficient and productive. The move toward standardization, efficiency and productivity in health care thus separates health occupations and creates a greater degree of dependence for health-care workers.

This increase in the division of labour is not unique to health care but is part of our general social development (Ehrenreich and Ehrenreich 1973 and 1975). Braverman (1974), in his analysis of work, shows that the separation of tasks that comes with increasing division of labour is not inevitable, but is part of a specific type of industrial development which destroys and de-skills occupational groups. The tasks of patient care, for example, are broken down into particular elements and standardized, so that patients with similar problems get similar care. Each task is accomplished by a particular occupational group.

The move to standardization in health-care work and patient care is supported by the ideals of efficiency and greater economic productivity.[2] For example, the move to greater economic efficiency with systems of patient classification is affecting Canadian nursing. Patient classification is seen to help efficiency by defining the care needed for a specific problem. However, classification doesn't allow for the individual differences patients exhibit. For example, establishing an average length of stay for a given illness leads to pressure for all patients to stay only that long in hospital, regardless of how well they have recovered. Objective decision-making is replacing traditional methods of practice in Canadian hospitals.

The standardization of patient illnesses is a process of classifying certain types of illnesses in terms of how much and what types of care and treatment the patient needs. This process takes away the nurse's control over decisions about care. The patient, as a result, is no longer seen as a particular patient with specific needs, but as only one of a group of patients with those needs. This objectification of the patient reduces the nurse's ability to make on-the-spot decisions about care.

Not only is control removed; the skill of the nurse in assessing patient needs decreases, since the nurse is no longer responsible for this task. When patient objectification takes place at the same time as increasing demands on the nurses' time, it is clear that the care given by nurses is threatened. Since the wellness of the patient in hospital involves more than undergoing medical procedures, more attention should be given to care (assurance, explanations, information and attention), and the control over this care should remain in the hands of the primary care-givers – nurses. Even though productivity may increase with objective methods, the costs are high.

An added oppression of female health-care workers is disguised within the ideals of professionalism in which the guiding principle is efficiency and productivity. These pressures place every nurse in a position of stress. This stress arises from three sources: the physician's orders for patient care, the hospital administrator's orders to reduce costs and be more efficient, and the patient's demands for care and attention. These pressures seem to increase with the size of the institution. If there is a shortage of nurses in large urban hospitals, it is not because there are too few nurses, but because nurses, in increasing numbers, are refusing to work full-time.[3] The lack of income, prestige and autonomy in their work has forced them to take a serious look at the demands placed on them. A further concern of nurses, a majority of whom are female, is their lack of control over their work in the male-dominated milieu of the hospital (Cleland 1971).

The increase in the division of medical labour creates some interesting effects: (1) it makes the different occupations dependent upon one another; (2) it has created a hierarchy of tasks and power, with physicians at the top; (3) it institutionalizes a specific knowledge within education, nursing and medical schools; and (4) it creates a monopoly over certain tasks and develops boundaries which, in many instances, cannot be crossed without problems (Ghan and Road 1971).

Professional groups must obtain a license or certificate to practise. Their qualifications enable them to justify practising a specific occupation which can be regulated by the state or their professional association. Thus, nurses are not permitted to do the tasks of doctors, even though they may be able to.[4] In practice, the tasks and definition of nursing are becoming increasingly cloudy, and it is difficult to separate nurses' specific knowledge and duties from those above and below them in the medical hierarchy. As Evans (1984, 115) states, "boundaries observed in any system are to a considerable extent arbitrary [and therefore] questions of jurisdiction will often arise."

If we assume that the social order we now have is the "best of all possible worlds" in which professionals are working in the best interests of all, then we can see increased dependence on professional control as beneficial. But if we do not assume that the professional elite is working in our best interests, then we perceive that the increased division of labour only subverts attempts to develop a universally beneficial health-care system, and alienates those working in it. The increased division of labour and the increased dependence and de-skilling of the health labour force actually decrease our ability to challenge the basic principles of medical practice. Thus, the dominance of scientific medicine has become stronger.

> Physicians have a professional monopoly of medical practice. They have the exclusive state-supported right, manifested in the "licensing" of physicians, to medical practice. With their licenses, physicians can legally do what no one else can, including cutting into the human body and prescribing drugs. (Conrad and Kern 1986, 123)

In Canada, this monopoly is further supported by a fee-for-service system by which the state guarantees the payment of medical costs.

Physicians

Within the Canadian health-care system, physicians are the primary group and nurses are their helpers. In a sense, physicians *are* the medical profession, and their task is to coordinate all health occupations in providing health care to their patients. Besides having the ability to influence those under them, physicians define and organize medical practice, and all other health workers are dependent upon their decisions.

Physicians make up 6.4% of the total health labour force (Canada 1971) and under their control there are the specialized occupations listed in Table 5.1 which lend support to the practice of medicine. Not all physicians have the same status; there are rankings which separate physicians on the basis of training, knowledge, power and income (Shapiro 1978, 81-101). Coates (1969), using the example of psychiatry, goes further by suggesting that a power elite or small controlling group exists within the Canadian medical profession. This group controls the professional medical organizations which dictate policy for the profession.

In 1981 there were more than 45,000 licensed physicians practising in Canada, or approximately one physician for every 538 Canadians (*Canada Year Book* 1985, 94). The number of physicians continues to grow, while the ratio between doctor and patient continues to fall, as shown in Table 5.2. (This is also true for nurses.)

TABLE 5.2

POPULATION PER PHYSICIAN, 1901-1981

Year	Population
1901	987
1911	970
1921	1,008
1931	1,034
1941	969
1951	977
1962	799
1971	659
1981*	538

SOURCE: Adapted from R. Hamowy, *Canadian Medicine: A Study in Restricted Entry.*
Toronto: The Fraser Institute, 1984. P. 270.
Canada Year Book 1985. P. 94.

In the ten-year period immediately after the introduction of medi-care in 1970, the number of physicians, interns and residents grew by 38% while the population grew by only 12.8%. Many experts, including the World Health Organization, have argued that Canada has a 10% surplus of general practitioners (Fairfax 1982, 14).[5] However, this aggre-gate number is a poor indicator of the supply: physicians can practise whereever they please, so that some provinces have greater rates of physicians per 100,000 population, while many rural areas in Canada are without physicians. There is a shortage of some specialties in many areas and acute cases may be far from medical care. Since many areas are without physicians, some provincial governments (Alberta, British Co-lumbia and Manitoba) are considering restricting the number of billing numbers they issue to practising physicians. They may also require physi-cians to work in under-served areas if they want a billing number (McKinley 1987; Silversides 1987a).[6]

Income and Workload

Since physicians are the highest-paid professional group in Canada (Allentuck 1978) there is controversy over why they are paid so much and, in times of economic restraint, why they are continually being paid many times the average wage. In response to doctors' increasing de-mands for more money, many provincial governments argue that physi-cians' fee increases should be subject to the same budget limits as other government employees. According to Fairfax (1982, 27), governments in

1982 were having a hard time dealing with fee increases of 10.5% in Manitoba and 26% in B.C. In early 1987 physicians were awarded a 5.6% fee increase in Manitoba ($10 million). In Alberta in 1987 the provincial government was talking about reducing payments to physicians or limiting the number of billing numbers.

In the summer of 1986 the physicians of Ontario organized a strike[7] to protest the government's elimination of extra-billing. This strike is an example of the consistent pressure exerted by physicians to control their right to extra-bill.[8] Many provincial governments will offer physicians fee increases to keep them from extra-billing. *The Globe and Mail* (11 February 1987) reported that even after legislation in Ontario prohibiting the practice, physicians still extra-bill. These extra charges are now labelled "administrative costs." Women in many Toronto hospitals are being charged a "stand-by" fee of $500 to ensure that an obstetrician will be on hand when their baby is born.[9] Implicit in these extra charges is the assumption that physicians are worth more and should be paid more (Owens 1983). *The Globe and Mail* also reported that when physicians feel an income squeeze they increase the volume of their billings. It is almost impossible for other professional groups to do this.

Both provincial governments and the Canadian population are concerned about reports that some physicians are being paid (at the time this book is being written) over $100,000 per year, while, "The National Council of Welfare estimated that in 1981 one Canadian family in eight was living below the poverty line" (Czerny and Swift 1984, 60). The Canadian Council on Social Development (1984, 58) estimates that 25.7% of households are below the poverty line. In 1985 the average after-tax income of physicians in Canada was over $63,000, while the average after-tax income of all working Canadians was $15,000 (Taylor, Stevenson and Williams 1984, 104). The average income of physicians, after expenses, rose from 3.26 to 5.57 times the average Canadian's income during the period 1946-1971 (Evans 1984, 15). Also, when unemployment was rising in Canada (to 7.4% in 1980 and 10.5% in 1984) there were no unemployed physicians (Canada 1985b, 70).[10] Table 5.3 shows the average gross income of physicians by province in 1985.

Over 50% of Canadian physicians are paid only on a fee-for-service basis, but the number of those who receive either all or part of their income as capitation, or salary, is increasing. Those physicians paid on a fee-for-service basis are the highest income earners and also the most conservative (Taylor, Stevenson and Williams 1984).

Physicians continually complain about not being paid enough and compare themselves to other professionals such as lawyers, dentists and professors. General income data, as shown in Figure 5.1 and Table 5.4, seem to support the argument that physicians are losing ground.

However, physicians experienced a great increase in their incomes with the introduction of medicare in 1962.

> The introduction of universal medical insurance was associated with immediate increases in average net physician earnings in seven of the ten provinces. A trend of rising medical incomes relative to the national average of wages and salaries, established in the 1950s, was therefore sustained in the 1960s. (Naylor 1986, 248)

TABLE 5.3

PHYSICIANS' AVERAGE GROSS INCOME BY PROVINCE, 1985

Province	Number of Physicians	Average Income
Newfoundland	400	$89,000
PEI	142	77,423
Nova Scotia	1,107	93,328
New Brunswick	610	96,577
Quebec	9,271	76,028
Ontario	11,736	95,711
Manitoba	1,458	92,452
Saskatchewan	1,089	80,067
Alberta	1,351	97,345
British Columbia	4,122	96,443
Yukon	15	59,307
NWT	30	61,130

SOURCE: Adapted from *Taxation Returns by Province and Occupation.* Catalogue 44, Table 8. Ottawa: Revenue Canada, 1985.

TABLE 5.4

A COMPARISON OF DOCTORS' INCOMES WITH THE INCOMES OF SELECTED GROUPS: 1967, 1971 AND 1977 (DOCTORS' INCOMES = 100%)

Year	Doctors	Dentists	Lawyers/ Notaries	Employees
1967	100	67.0	79.6	17.2
1972	100	68.7	73.0	16.7
1977	100	84.3	81.8	24.1

SOURCE: E. Black, "Dealing with the Doctors: The Canadian Experience." *Monthly Review* Sept. 1981. P. 32. Copyright © 1978 by John Ehrenreich. Reprinted by permission.

FIGURE 5.1

PHYSICIANS' EARNINGS COMPARED WITH OTHER PROFESSIONAL INCOMES AND AVERAGE WAGES

Indices of

(A)   Average net earnings from all sources of self-employed Canadian Physicians;
(B)   Weighted average net earnings from all sources of self-employed Lawyers, Dentists, Accountants, Engineers and Architects;
(C)   Average weekly wages and salaries (Industrial composite);
(D)   Consumer price index, all items.

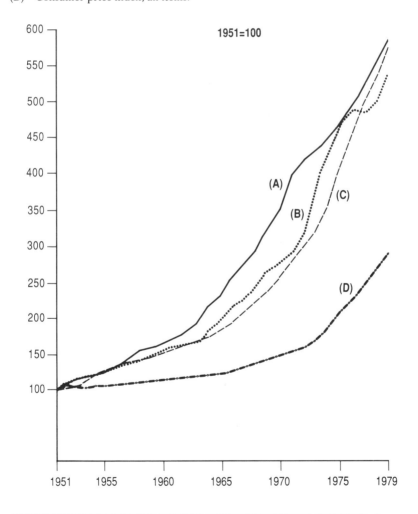

SOURCE: M. Fairfax, "Canada: Higher Fees, Lower Wages." *Health/Pac Bulletin* 13, no. 4. P. 15.

Naylor goes on to say that while physicians' incomes had been 3.7 times the national average in 1950, they rose to 4.85 times the national average in the 1960s, and to 5.4 times the national average in 1971. (Fairfax (1982, 15) argues that physicians' earnings "went from 4.8 times the industrial average in 1961 to 6.5 times in 1971.") (The national average includes all wages; the industrial average includes only the industrial sector of the economy.) But by 1978 this figure had declined to 3.4, and physicians reacted by pressuring federal and provincial governments to increase their fee schedules. Naylor points out that the decrease in physicians' incomes was due more to transformations within the profession, such as the increase in specialization and in numbers of physicians, than to a decrease in fees.

Doctors in Canada have an advantage, since the introduction of a national health care system (medicare), in that they are guaranteed payment of their bills by the provincial governments. This is not the case for physicians in the United States, or for any other business person in Canada. Lawyers' fees, for example, are paid directly by the client.

Yet physicians perceive themselves as relatively deprived in relation to other professional groups and their medical colleagues. One study (Taylor, Stevenson and Williams 1984) found that physicians, both general practitioners and specialists, thought that they should be getting approximately $17,500 more than they are now getting. Many physicians consider it their right to charge what they feel they are worth, and to try to increase their incomes by holding onto the right to extra-bill or increase the numbers of patients they see per week. This move is aimed not only at increasing income, but also at maintaining control over their working situation.

Hospital administrators, provincial governments and patients alike are now questioning whether higher paid health is better health, and whether more money gives physicians a greater incentive. On the other hand, people who treat health as a commodity assume that the best physicians should be paid the most and that specialists should demand higher fee schedules.

Physicians tend to justify their large incomes in three ways: (1) they have to undergo extensive training; (2) they have a shortened period of lifetime earnings because of their late entry into the work force; and (3) they work long hours in conditions of stress. There is also the belief that physicians are somehow a special group, set apart from other professional groups.

All the above arguments can be disputed. First, even though physicians undergo extensive training in Canada, their education is subsidized to a large extent by provincial governments. As well, physicians spend less time than do Ph.D.s and research scientists in training for their profession. Second, doctors are not the only professionals who enter the work force in their late twenties. Third, most occupations have large amounts of stress, and it is self-serving on the part of physicians to claim that only they make critical life decisions. All professionals do so when working with people.

Physicians' workloads are also an issue of debate since physicians' incomes, if they are not on salary, are tied to the number of patients they see (Wolfe and Badgley 1973). "The fee-for-service remuneration scheme permitted doctors to continue controlling their personal earnings (with payment guaranteed by government) by upping the level of services rendered" (Fairfax 1982, 14). That is, physicians can increase their incomes by increasing the number of patients they see, or they can charge for services which are not necessary and may even be harmful. This practice encourages the overservicing of patients (Black 1981, 34).

According to Taylor, Stevenson and Williams (1984, 115), physicians say they work approximately 49 hours per week and are on call approximately 28 hours per week. On average, practitioners see 136 patients per week and specialists see 76.2 patients per week. Many other professionals work as many hours as physicians; however, physicians can control the amount of work they take on. Since the introduction of medicare there has been a drop in weekly hours worked (Fairfax 1982, 15). Many argue, and statistics tend to back them up, that each year physicians are increasing the numbers of patients they see. This increases their income and decreases the amount of time spent with each patient. It is also argued that the fee-for-service system has a built-in economic incentive to reduce the quality of care and rely on quick remedies, especially drugs, while ignoring the time-consuming aspects of patient education.

Another way Canadian physicians increase their earnings is by shifting costs to hospitals. Canada's system of provincially funded hospitalization plans "encourages doctors to reduce their own office overhead and increase the hourly number of income generating visits by evaluating their patients in an institution paid for by public funds" (Fairfax 1982, 15).

Physicians, as opposed to the majority of Canadians, can work as much or as little as they want and when they want, therefore it is easier for them to control their income than for other professional groups. Also, since physicians are seen by the government as independent business executives, they can retire when they want and are entitled to various tax benefits that salaried professionals cannot claim. There is also a funded institutional structure, the hospital, which supports the work of physicians.

However, the need for financial restraint in health care is challenging the independent position of the physician. The current attempts by the medical profession to control its own destiny reflect a concern over the possible loss of professional autonomy. Discussions of workload and income are secondary to the issue of autonomy.

The Proletarianization of Doctors

Since the publication of the Lalonde Report in 1974, there has been a general realization that the cost of medicine is rising. However, there is considerable debate over the possible solutions to this problem. The argument is being shaped in certain ways by the medical profession; in debates over funding and control, physicians always use the fear of illness as their trump card, and claim that more money means better health. There is no evidence to support this claim, and various groups in Canada are arguing for a transformation in the practice of health care to reduce costs.

One group, the Fraser Institute, is arguing for a reprivatization of medical practice which would bring competition back to medicine (Blomquist 1979). The reprivatization of medical care which is currently developing in Britain is also gaining support among Canadian physicians (Weller 1983). In the United States big business is moving into health care, arguing that it can reduce costs by better management. In Canada, governments and social agencies are arguing for the elimination of the physician's dominance and the fee-for-service system (Hancock 1986), thereby placing the physician directly under the control of the government. This government control, ideally, would lead to a more efficient system of medical practice. In some sense, both groups argue for economic efficiency without a reduction in the population's health. Both moves would have grave consequences for physicians since they would have to lose their independence, to business in the U.S., and to government in Britain.

The introduction of government health insurance and the intrusion of business in medicine in Canada, as well as in Britain and the U.S., have resulted in a loss of power, status, autonomy and control for the medical profession. Through the degradation and the de-skilling of their work, physicians, along with other health-care workers, ". . . are losing influence and autonomy in their work and becoming more like alienated factory workers" (Wahn 1987, 422). An increase in the division of labour in medical practice limits the knowledge and skill that any given physician is capable of, thereby reducing his ability to be a general practitioner. That is, by becoming more skilled in a specific aspect of medical practice, physicians are becoming de-skilled in general medical practice. Thus, Black (1981, 32) states that the medical profession is becoming proletarianized: it is gradually losing its autonomy and control and doctors are becoming salaried workers for either government or business.

Many physicians in the United States are employed by large corporate hospitals organized on the principles of profit-making corporations, for example the Humana Institute. In Britain, physicians are salaried employees of the state but are allowed to bill private patients on the side.[11] In Canada, even though provincial governments fund fee-for-service medicine and administer most hospitals, physicians are still able to control their private practices. Evans (1984, 141) points out that in Canada, provincial governments determine the numbers of places available in medical practice, the number of spaces in medical school and the number of billing numbers, and therefore the medical profession does not have an absolute monopoly.

The development of medical markets and bureaucracies in the past 100 years has changed the practice of medicine and the relations between doctor and patient (Larson 1977). The pressure that is being put upon provincial governments by the medical associations of Canada for the right to extra-bill or control some part of the billing process can be seen as the struggle of the profession against the trend toward the loss of autonomy and control, or proletarianization. The consequences of this process of proletarianization would be (1) the loss of control over non-health-related issues and where, when, and how long physicians will practise; (2) a greater regulation of work routine; and (3) standardization of practice and procedures. Starr (1982, 446) argues that even though this process is occurring, ". . . the total loss of control over the conditions of work as well as a severe reduction in compensation" is not likely to happen. The health-care system requires the full participation of the medical profession and the definitions of health continue to be in the hands of physicians even though physicians ". . . are experiencing forms of economic and organizational alienation" (Wahn 1987, 436).

Even though the medical profession is coming under more regulation by governments because of the rising costs of health care, and although the organization and general working conditions of physicians are changing, in Canada the profession still controls the definition of health and illness. In some areas it still retains absolute control: (1) content and standards of education, (2) licensing of physicians, (3) legal regulations, and (4) evaluation procedures (Goode 1960, 903). However, even these powers may be eroded in the future.

On the other hand, Canada differs from the United States in that there is a legal constraint to the takeover of medical practice by big business in Canada. "Canadian licensure laws in medicine and dentistry prohibit the ownership of any part of a practice by anyone other than a licensed member of the profession" (Evans 1984, 115). Therefore, even though Canada's provincial governments are gradually reducing the medical monopoly, they are ensuring a degree of monopoly for physicians.

Nurses

Conflicting Demands

Nurses form the largest health occupational group. Nursing can be called a para-profession since nurses must act as professionals yet they have little autonomy or control over their working situation (Coburn 1987, 457-60). Nursing, following the lead of the medical profession, is attempting to professionalize itself but cannot because it is not independent. Even though nursing has its own sphere of expertise (patient care, especially the psycho-social aspects), there is an obedience to hospital and physician authority (Hofling 1966). In fact, the role of the nurse closely follows the traditional stereotyped role of the female: ". . . a woman serves sacrifically, and supports and protects a dominant male" (Reeder and Mauksch 1979, 216).

Nurses have their own schools and curricula, and their own code of ethics, professional organizations and licensing qualifications. The focus of their education should be different from that of medical training. However, the increased encouragement to be health-care *professionals* means a continued emphasis on science in their training, instead of on interactive patient care. This is obvious from the curricula for the Nurse Baccalaureate programs in Canada. There is an increasing emphasis on physiology, microbiology and statistics. This focus on science blurs the line between the roles of nurse and physician, and nurses who attempt to maintain an autonomous area of expertise are frustrated in their attempts.[12]

The training of nurses also contributes to frustrations in their practice in other ways as well. First, although nurses have control over their education, this education cannot be separated from the general focus of medical care. Second, nurses are taught to leave behind their human qualities and take on "professional" attitudes, yet they are constantly called upon to be the "human face" of medicine in patient care. These contradictory demands can result in "burnout" (Fawzy 1981 and Gray-Toft and Anderson 1981) and general dissatisfaction with nursing jobs (Godfrey 1978).[13]

Nurses are also in the middle of the doctor/patient relationship within the hospital and in other health-care settings (Millman 1977). Nursing is considered to focus on the quality of patient care and the patient's psycho-social needs. Nurses thus are torn between wanting to be empathetic toward their patients and wanting to be detached, professional care-givers.

Duff and Hollingshead (1968) state that the focus of nursing is changing from the patient to task performance. "Nursing facilities have tended to insist on students viewing their patients objectively, which has operated to deemphasise an intimate nurse/patient relationship" (Cockerham 1986, 191). In this view, a good nurse is one who completes her tasks, not one who spends time with patients.

Recently in Manitoba there has been a move to upgrade nursing by requiring all nurses to have a Bachelor of Nursing degree, which requires two years of study after the RN, by the year 2000. (It is interesting that the now-defunct nurse-practitioner program was a three-year program.) BN programs take three or four years and include a two-year RN program. This trend to higher educational requirements is well developed in the U.S. and is putting pressure on nurses to return to school or stay in school longer. However, extra education takes more time out of a nurse's working life without promising higher rewards for the effort. Also, the addition of another level of qualification creates divisions and competition within nursing. The upgrading of nursing education will not necessarily lead to more autonomy or responsibility for nurses, but may introduce them to a greater scope of medical care without the rewards.

The practice of nursing is also becoming more complicated. Many physicians are pressuring nurses to do tasks which should be their own responsibility, for example informing a patient that she is dying. Financial pressures will probably lead to nurses being trained in time-consuming procedures such as patient education, which physicians want to avoid. Some physicians in the United States and Canada favour the return of the nurse-midwife because of the high insurance rates required for obstetricians. This move is also favoured by governments since nurse-midwives are less costly than physicians who do the same techniques.

Status and Income

Today, there is a trend to viewing the nurse as a physician's co-worker and team member. However, a number of researchers show that the nurse is still a subordinate to the physician (Bates 1978) and must abide by specific rules of interaction, as in the "Doctor-Nurse Game" (Stein 1967). Reeder and Mauksch (1979, 215) say that there is evidence to suggest that those entering nursing express a desire to serve their doctors just as much as their patients.

The subordinate role of nurses can also be seen in their income in relation to physicians'. Nurses are paid, on average, 21% less than physicians, as shown in Table 5.5.

TABLE 5.5

NURSES' INCOMES AS A PERCENTAGE OF PHYSICIANS' INCOMES (FULL-TIME INCOMES)

Year	Percent of Physician's Income
1962	22%
1966	20%
1972	19%
1982*	23%

SOURCE: M. Swartz, "The Politics of Reform: Conflict and Accommodation in Canadian Health Policy." In L. Panitch (ed.), *The Canadian State*. Toronto: U. of Toronto Press, 1977. P. 332.

*1982 is for Manitoba only.

The income gap between doctors and nurses increased between 1962 and 1972, as shown in Table 5.6, but the gap is gradually closing in the 1980s as the rate of increase in physicians' incomes diminishes.

TABLE 5.6
INCOME TRENDS WITHIN THE HEALTH CARE SECTOR, 1962-72

	Income			Income increase	
	1962	1966	1972	1962-72	1966-72
Selected hospital workers[a]					
Registered nurse	$3744/yr	4668	7656	104%	64%
Nursing auxiliary	2592	3312	5760	122	74
X-ray technician (male)	4092	4728	7644	87	62
Maid	1932	2628	4560	130	74
Hospital executives[b]					
Chief executive officer		$13,500/yr	$24,000/yr		69%
Assistant to CEO		10,250	15,000		54
Chief financial officer		9750	14,000		47
Chief nursing		9000	14,000		58
Physicians[c]					
All fee-practice MD	$16,966/yr	$23,262	$39,977	136%	72%

SOURCE: M. Swartz, "The Politics of Reform: Conflict and Accommodation in Canadian Health Policy." In L. Panitch (ed.), *The Canadian State.* Toronto: U. of Toronto Press, 1977. P. 332.

[a] Computed from monthly salary data, assuming 12 months employment. Nurses were selected because they are the largest group of hospital workers, and maids because they won the largest pay increases among hospital workers. X-ray technicians' pay increases were typical of those won by technical support staff. Source: Health and Welfare Canada, *Salaries and Wages in Canadian Hospitals, 1962-1970* and *1969-73*
[b] These figures consist of an unweighted average of the annual salaries of these executives in hospitals of 500+ beds and 100-199 beds. Both salaries and changes in salary varied widely by hospital size but these figures provide a good illustration for comparative purposes. Data are not available for 1962. Source: as above
[c] Source: published and unpublished statistics provided by Health and Welfare Canada. The figures reflect net income from medical services, where net income is income after office/practice expenses but before taxes. As with all businessmen, some percentage of deductions from gross income are recovered in the future (sale of equipment, goodwill) and so the actual figures are underestimates. The discrepancy has apparently grown over time as physicians have increasingly utilized accountants, management consultants, etc.

Other factors which influence the relationship between doctors and nurses are: (1) gender, (2) age and (3) social class. Even though more women are becoming physicians, more men are not becoming nurses; nursing continues to be a female occupation. Nurses tend to be young because of the shift work, stress and lack of possibilities for advancement (Moccia 1982). (That is, as they get older they drop out.) Also, the class background of nurses continues to be lower than that of physicians, who come from professional families (Shapiro 1978, 14; Reeder and Mauksch 1979, 215). For many, nursing is not a full-time career because of the lack of opportunities for advancement, save in teaching and administration. Nursing is becoming a part-time job for women who supplement their family's income in this way. The decision to work part-time can be the result of other factors as well. Not only is the job highly stressful, women can often get better pay working in retail sales, for example, and may be drawn away from nursing. The lack of income and sufficient career options, along with family demands, lead many women to abandon nursing.

The questions of what it means to be part of a professional group and to act as a professional have been debated in sociology for a long time. These debates are significant since they allow us to understand the past, present and future developments of professional groups, and how an occupation like nursing may never be able to be a profession, since it cannot separate itself from the dominance of the medical profession and reflects gender relations within Canadian society.

Models of Professionalism

In Western societies there is a mystique associated with the label "professional." The term has taken on many meanings such as "expert," "sophisticated," "well-educated," "independent" and "dedicated." The term is often used loosely, as in "the oldest profession," "professional thief" and "call the professional." The label "professional" becomes useless, however, if it can be applied to any type of work; not everyone is a professional. Many occupational groups call themselves a profession in an attempt to "flatter themselves or try to persuade others of their importance" (Friedson 1970, 4). "Everett Hughes [a noted sociologist] describes professionals as those who profess to know better than others the nature of certain affairs" (Mumford 1983, 249).

Though there may be some debate over the status of many occupations, it is fairly certain that medicine can be called a profession.

It should be clear that it would be folly to be dogmatic about any definition of "profession" or to assume that its definition is so well known that it warrants no discussion . . . if anything "is" a profession, it is contemporary medicine. (Friedson 1970, 4)

But is nursing a profession? Nurses are constantly told by their teachers to act like professionals, as though there were certain qualities a person must exhibit in order to be professional. In this view, professionalism is "... defined as a set of attributes said to be characteristic of professionals" (Friedson 1970, 70). The training of the professional should instill an impersonal attitude, and "professional" acts should be independent of personal interest (Friedson 1986, 147). Being a professional means to inspire confidence and trust in the professional/client relationship. Thus, to be unprofessional is to be untrustworthy, according to this definition.

In sociology there is some debate as to what makes a profession different from an occupation. Some (Johnson 1972, 13-14; Blane 1982, 213-14), following Durkheim's concept of altruism, make the distinction between a profession and an occupation according to whether the job involves dealing with people or things; if it deals with things it is an occupation, and if it deals with people, it is a profession. Since there is no word analogous to "professional" for those working in non-professional occupations, it may be assumed that we attribute certain personal characteristics to professionals because of the work they do. Professionals are thought to adhere to the notion of the "common good" and to set an example of moral behaviour, as in "acting like a professional."

Sociology uses two basic models to try to understand professionalization (the process of becoming a profession) and the relations between professionals and their clients. These models enable us to distinguish between professions and occupations, and demonstrate why professions are given high status in our society. The first model, trait theory, looks at the qualities or characteristics of the professional. The second model, which can be called relational theory, looks at the interaction within practitioner/client relationships. The first builds upon the unique attributes of professionalism while the second builds on the control of the service and the client.

Characteristics of a Profession: Trait Theory

Trait theory focuses on the qualities which the professional as an individual and the profession as a group possess. These qualities, usually defined by the professionals themselves, are considered to have been acquired by the specific group in its efforts to move from the status of a trade to that of a profession (Coe 1978, 200-201). Box 5.1 shows Mumford's (1983, 250-51) list of eleven attributes associated with professions.

Box 5.1

ATTRIBUTES ASSOCIATED WITH PROFESSIONS

1. The hallmark of the most firmly established professions is that they require for membership a prolonged and specialized training in a body of abstract knowledge. Such training provides the setting in which new recruits can be socialized as well as trained to join the profession.
2. Professionals characteristically report a relatively high degree of work satisfaction compared with nonprofessionals. Few people voluntarily leave a profession, and a relatively high proportion claim that if they had it to do over again, they would choose the same work.
3. A highly developed ethic or rhetoric and a shared perspective that includes the idea of a service orientation support the profession's claim for the importance of its services and justify its exclusive right to provide those services.
4. Professionals believe their work is special and worthy of esteem and protection. Nonprofessionals tend to accord the professional special prestige.
5. Members of a profession tend to feel a sense of identity and solidarity with fellow professionals.
6. The profession is able to exert some social control over members. Professions tend to be taken as reference groups by members, who learn to care more about what a colleague thinks of them than about what an outsider might think.
7. The profession is able to offer members some protection against nonprofessionals.
8. The profession limits admission and controls education and training of its own. This control over access is often mandated by the society.
9. The profession is able to exert control over licensing. The most highly developed professions are able to enlist the government in protecting the right of members to be the exclusive providers of services designated as the profession's own. In medicine, physicians sit on state licensing boards, and legal action can be taken against anyone who provides services without a license.
10. The profession commands autonomy for itself and sometimes zealously fights any threat to its autonomy. Members of all occupations try to protect themselves against excessive surveillance by outsiders, but professionals characteristically are particularly successful in this protection and extremely sensitive to any threat to their autonomy.
11. Members of the profession can command high prestige, power, and income.

One of the problems with the trait theory is that it offers no way to understand the relation between the particular characteristics of each professional and the relationship between the professional and a client. It also assumes that any person who is a professional will have these attributes and that these attributes will be uniform throughout the profession. There is a further assumption that these professional attributes will force the professional to act in the best interests of the client or patient. This assumption has been shown to be without foundation. Some professionals will act this way, but not all professionals must or will act that way.

> To take one example, the view that the profession of law mediates between the power of the state and the needs of the individual citizen is often expressed as a form of altruism whereby the lawyer is regarded as the guardian of the rule of law for the benefit of all. The profession's vested interest in a given legal order renders its services irrelevant to those groups in the society who seek radical change in the existing order. (Johnson 1972, 25)

Johnson's perspective can be applied to the medical profession and trait theory. That is, physicians are the protectors of the medical system, and they have a vested interest in perpetuating their position. Should we assume then that they are acting in our best interests?

Practitioner / Client Relations: Relational Theory

Within the health-care system physicians are dominant; it is they who, as a group, shape the goals and models of medical practice (Coburn and Biggs 1987, 378-80). Johnson (1972) argues that in order to understand the differences between occupations and professions, focus must centre on the power and control professionals have over their clients. If the practitioner is able to impose his definitions upon the situation and client, then the practitioner has professional control. For Johnson, an occupational group must have three available sources of power in order to become and maintain itself as a profession. In the case of the Canadian medical profession these all apply since, in some sense, physicians are the controllers or producers of health care, and their patients or consumers are dependent upon them. (It is difficult to speak of this relation without using the terms "producer" and "consumer"; however, this is a special kind of producer/consumer relationship.)

> (1) The esoteric character of the knowledge used by the specialist is a power resource, because it produces variations in the degree of uncertainty of the consumer-producer relationship and the potential for autonomy of the practitioner.
> (2) The amount of social power which the occupation group membership has outside the occupation, such as also being members of a dominant class or caste in the society.
> (3) Characteristics of the consumer – the "social composition and character of the source of demand" – specifically, the larger, more heterogeneous and fragmented the consumers, the more easily the producers may impose their definitions of the situation upon the consumer. (Marsden 1977, 5)

There is a power relationship not only between physicians and their patients but also within the medical profession. Within the profession, medical educators (Marsden 1977) and executive members of the medical associations (Taylor, Stevenson and Williams 1984) set the values and purposes of the profession and can be referred to as an elite group (Coates 1969). The beliefs and values of individual professionals are not necessarily the same as the beliefs and values of the profession. Not all physicians are members of professional organizations, such as the Canadian Medical Association and the various provincial medical associations,[14] and many physicians may be opposed to the profession's stand on certain issues, for example free access to abortion. Friedson (1970) shows that physicians are more concerned with external pressures to their authority than with the enforcing of conformity within the profession.

Examples of pressure to keep control and power in the profession can be seen in some recent events concerning Dr. Henry Morgentaler. It can be argued that the various medical associations were not disturbed by the fact that Morgentaler was providing abortions, but were concerned that he was doing it outside the institutions of medicine (hospitals) and bypassing the abortion committees of doctors who regulate who is to receive an abortion.

Medicine is not only a profession, it is a set of social institutions which have rules governing behaviours within clinics, medical schools and hospitals. These institutions set the rights and privileges of the various members of the medical profession. Physicians who practise outside the medical boundaries are as much a threat to medical dominance as are practising lay midwives who have no medical training. This has historically been the case when a group is labelled as "quacks."

> Charlatanism and quackery are a creation of professionalism and not the cause of it. That is to say that periods in which it is claimed that charlatanism is rife and needs to be stamped out are just those periods when an occupation is attempting to establish or struggling to maintain a monopolistic position. Practice can be unqualified only where a monopoly of skill by one group exists. (Johnson 1972, 57)

Even though there is evidence to suggest that the power of the medical profession is declining (Black 1981; Wahn 1987; Coburn and Biggs 1987), physicians no longer have to fight to establish their particular view of medicine since it has become not only part of our legal system but also part of our everyday consciousness. Though physicians may be on the road to proletarianization, their definition of health and the types of medicine to be used are not in any danger.

As a professional group, physicians maintain control over the practice of medicine in Canada by controlling their patients and colleagues. Marsden (1974 and 1977) uses Johnson's model to elaborate on the Ontario medical profession and outlines professional control within medicine in four points (Marsden 1974, 13-20).

(1) *Social Distance*
There has been a rapidly increasing division of labour and interdependence within
the medical profession evidenced by the increasing number and variety of both fields
of specialization and organizational settings for practice. With this increase in specialization, social distance between doctors has increased and each less specialized
person is more dependent upon each more specialized person for information.

(2) *Science*
There is another type of power . . . this is the relation of contemporary medical
practice to the ideology and social institutions of science. [The] exclusive access to
doing science as well as the formal credentials of educators as a group is one base of
power which the educator-researcher group are able to draw upon in order to
support their definition of the producer-client relationship.

(3) *Education*
If colleague control works at all, it assuredly works in a setting where the doctors'
procedures are subject to the critical view of medical students and colleagues daily.
There is no possibility in the teaching-researching situation for . . . normative
relaxation.

(4) *Social Class*
Doctors in Ontario tend to come from high social class backgrounds. Within the
medical profession doctors . . . who teach and research are predominantly a select
group drawn from the dominant groups in social class structure.

The place of the medical profession within the larger social structure
supports their privileged position in our society. Physicians are the highest paid profession and are a homogeneous group in terms of ethnicity,
class background and education. Also, socialization, medical school, class
background and residency all tend to inculcate members of the profession with a particular set of values, beliefs and attitudes. This view says
that physicians are concerned with controlling all aspects of health care
from recruitment to regulation. Friedson (1970), however, says that "the
demand for monopoly control of the profession by the profession may
have less to do with the corpus of specialized and technical knowledge of
medicine, which is used to justify this demand, than with effort to sustain
the position of power and status of physicians vis-à-vis other health
professionals and their patients" (Mishler 1981, 205).

The Development of the Medical Profession

In line with the two models outlined above, there are corresponding
models of the origins and development of professions as we know them
today. Although each model starts from the premise that professionalization began with industrial capitalism (following Durkheim or Marx) the
two models see the rise of professionalism differently.

Wilenksy (1964, 142-46), working in the tradition of trait theory,
outlines five stages in the natural history of a profession:

1) the emergence of a full time occupation; 2) the establishment of a training school;
3) the founding of a professional association; and 4) political agitation directed
towards the protection of the association by law; and 5) the adoption of a formal code.

This model gives an evolutionary view of the steps taken, in sequence, to secure the profession's position of control. Even though these steps seem to be a natural progression, from birth to full professional control, there is much more to the history of the medical profession in Canada, especially the drive for a self-serving monopoly.[15]

Hamowy (1984) studied the legal restrictions to entry into the Canadian medical practice and found that the inordinate amount of prestige, power and income afforded contemporary medicine has its roots in the 19th century. The medical profession in Canada, historically, has been self-serving. Its motive in restricting entry to the practice of medicine was not to protect the health of the population (by eliminating quacks), but to create a medical monopoly. Professions cannot accomplish this monopoly without the support of the government behind them. "As is usually the case with professions, state regulation of the Canadian medical services market came at the behest not of consumers but of practitioners" (Naylor 1986, 16).

The work of Hamowy and Naylor is supported by Larson (1977, 14). She states that the rise of professionalism is linked to the control over a market for a specific commodity, and in the case of medicine the commodity is health. "The 'great transformation' [the industrial revolution] presented the professional 'entrepreneurs' with expanding and 'free' markets." According to Larson (1977, 14) professionals had to do three things to gain control and thereby enforce their professional position:

(1) For the professional market to exist a "distinctive" commodity had to be produced; (2) For a secure market to arise, the superiority of one kind of service had to be clearly established with regard to competing products; and (3) At least a moderate guarantee that the recruits' educational investment would be protected had to be sought from the beginning.

This view states that in the creation of a professional monopoly over the medical market and the production of health as a commodity, the medical profession had to establish some credibility with the public and support from the government.

Physician Evaluation

Implicit in the medical profession's autonomy as a profession is that only physicians can evaluate the work of other physicians. Mumford (1983, 256-57) says that physicians can be detested by other physicians and still practise medicine. As well, since physicians work independently of one another, there is little association between work excellence as judged by other physicians and their actual work with patients. Some would argue that the medical licensing system and the set of review boards protect the public, and that ill patients are in no position to judge their physician. Mumford (1983, 257) outlines three criticisms against these assertions:

(1) For some aspects of patient care, the patient may be the best person to evaluate. Patients with chronic conditions become well informed about their illnesses and have the opportunity to observe and compare physician performance.

(2) If licenses are given once in a lifetime and are automatically renewable without further proof of soundness, skill or knowledge of latest advances, the public may not be protected by the licensing mechanism.

(3) Personal loyalty, friendship, or self-interest can also influence how physicians evaluate peers.

Often physicians do not take, or routinely fail, specialist exams, yet they continue to do the same specialized type of work. The only drawback is that they cannot call themselves specialists. Cockerham (1986, 172) says that what is important in the evaluation of medical practice is not the technical expertise or error of the physician but the moral principles behind the medical judgement.

Physicians argue that standards must be in their hands because they are the only ones able to judge medical competence and protect the public against unscrupulous practitioners or quacks. We might ask who protects the public from physicians. And how do we know whether other methods of medicine (say, homeopathy) are bad, or just competition for the dominance of scientific medicine. Physicians have in the past judged many practices (for example, acupuncture) as non-medical or harmful, and barred their practitioners from practice. However, once these methods have been accepted as having merit, then they are assumed under the practice of physicians.

Millman (1986, 334) analyzed a hospital mortality review where physicians had gathered to review the "question of whether the patient's death might have been avoided had the medical judgement been more sound . . . what is usually involved in these cases is a question of misdiagnosis or of appropriate medical action taken too late." Since the stakes are very high – a judgement of error means, at the least, ridicule, and at worst, a malpractice suit – the review functions to neutralize criticism and justify the physician's actions. "Flukes" or mistakes are often cited, however, the blame is focused on the patient. Ultimately, "the physician's errors are made to seem understandable and inconsequential in a life fated for disaster by the patient's own doing" (Millman 1986, 339). A "gentleman's agreement" exists among physicians to overlook their colleagues' mistakes (Cockerham 1986, 173).

The letters "MD" after a person's name are no guarantee that the person will not commit crimes or harm patients; it is not even a guarantee that the person will work in the best interests of patients.[16] Each province has a medical review board that polices abuses of patients and billing for certain medical procedures. Every year many physicians are brought before these boards and are forced to repay their respective health-care systems. However, only the glaring abuses are detected, and many abuses go unnoticed. Even though a physician may over-bill, and have to pay back a certain sum of money, his action is not seen as criminal and the offense will not restrict his practice. The courts cannot take away a physician's right to practise. Only medical review boards have the power to prohibit a physician from practising medicine, by taking away his license. Therefore, physicians who have abused the system or committed a crime may still be allowed to practise medicine.

It is not our intention to start a witch hunt for criminal doctors, but to point out our inability to deal with physicians' mistakes and show the need we have to develop a system of physician evaluation and accountability.

Information and Medical Language

Many physicians still believe that, in some instances, information about a patient's illness should be withheld from the patient (Waitzkin and Stoeckle 1976). Even if this belief is couched in the understanding that the information might do a patient more harm than good, as in the case of cancer, withholding information from a patient can only create stratified patterns of social relations between the doctor and the patient. This applies not only to information but also to the language in which that information is given. Although physicians may be willing to give information to the patient, they may do so in a language that is incomprehensible to the patient.

A technical language or medical discourse not only translates life's problems into special medical terms, but this language forms the basis of misunderstanding between the doctor and the patient (Mumford 1983, 216). The jargon, "medspeak," separates the medical profession from the public and creates an elite of those who can speak it. By using specialized medical terms the physician (1) withholds knowledge from the patient, (2) ensures a lack of intimacy with the patient, and (3) buffers himself from a barrage of questions.

The patient, many times confused by this, can only assume that the physician knows what he is talking about and that he is working in her best interest. Many times physicians are themselves confused by the medical jargon of their own colleagues. Technical language may be used to cloak the inexperience and incompetence of a physician (Hass and Shaffir 1978). Simplicity in communicating ideas to patients is not emphasized in medical education and has not been demanded by patients. However, the growing number of self-help groups are spurring interest in a more understandable communication between doctor and patient.

Medical Education

The type of education doctors receive is an important focus of study for those concerned with the quality of medicine practised in Canada. If we want better or different types of physicians, then there must be better or different medical education. There is research to show that the medical school does socialize students into the role of the medical professional (Hass and Shaffir 1978) but there is also evidence to show that the content of medical education has little relation to the practice of medicine (Shapiro 1978). Within medical schools, medical educators strive to transform the ways physicians are trained and to update the content of the training, which has been relatively stagnant since the 1910 Flexner Report[17] into medical education (Berliner 1975; Hudson 1978). However, education is difficult to change since it is institutionalized and since at times it reflects the ideals of medicine rather than the reality of medical practice.[18]

Canada has sixteen medical schools, which are all associated with a university. After two years of university, mainly in sciences, a student takes the MCAT exam (a standardized medical school entrance exam developed in the U.S.). In 1976 there were 8,079 applicants for medical school, and out of this group 5,223 were acceptable (i.e. had the required qualifications) and 1,804 were actually accepted. Eleven years later, in 1986, there were 7,832 applicants, of whom 1,746 were admitted (Ryten and Watanabe 1987).

Except for McMaster University, the four-year MD program consists of two years studying medicine and science and two more years in clinical experience. At McMaster, clinical experience starts almost immediately. After these four years, there is a year of internship and then residency (usually two years), an apprentice type of learning.

In 1982, 1,749 medical students graduated from medical school in Canada. The number of graduates has been on the rise since 1960 (Hamowy 1984, 276-77), as shown in Table 5.7. Recently, provincial governments have thought it necessary to control the number of medical school positions, in order to control the supply of doctors and reduce costs.

The purpose of medical education is to train and educate applicants and to maximize the chances that they will become respectable, skillful and knowledgeable practitioners. Hass and Shaffir (1978) say that medical education also trains the students to act, feel, speak and look like doctors, to develop a professional "cloak of competence." However, many skills which are needed in the practice of medicine are still not taught; it is assumed that medical students will "pick up" these skills in their interactions with other physicians and learn on the job. They are not taught how to manage doctor/patient interactions, generate patient cooperation, educate patients in nutrition and exercise, or deal with their own emotional feelings.

TABLE 5.7

GRADUATES OF CANADIAN MEDICAL SCHOOLS 1960-1980 (3-YEAR AVERAGES, AND GRADUATES PER 100,000 POPULATION)

Years	Graduates (Average)	Per 100,000 Population
1960-62	855	4.69
1963-65	878	4.55
1966-68	942	4.62
1969-71	1,087	5.10
1972-74	1,391	6.31
1975-77	1,642	7.17
1978-80	1,753	7.37

SOURCE: R. Hamowy, *Canadian Medicine: A Study in Restricted Entry.* Toronto: The Fraser Institute, 1984. P. 276-77.

In Canada, McMaster University is the focus of an experiment in the quality of medical education. This experiment is moving away from "hard science" in medical education to a more "patient-centred" approach. Harvard University in the U.S. has followed the lead of McMaster in attempting to ". . . help students understand and utilize the influence of family, society and culture in treating a patient's illness" (Wallace 1986, 23).

The main concern of medical students is passing their school and licensing exams in order to become physicians. Subjects in the curriculum which are not on their licensing exams, for example medical history, social science and humanities courses (which are supposed to make physicians more aware of the concerns of the patients they treat) are viewed as unimportant because they would use up valuable time that is needed to study for exams. Until now medical students have not had to have a B.A. to enter medical school. Therefore they have selected undergraduate courses that will allow them to keep their grade point average up, rather than to acquire an understanding of the world around them. This is also true in the U.S., where medical students must have a four-year liberal arts B.A. before entering medical school.

The medical student's concentration on passing exams, rather than understanding patients, is caused not by what is taught, but by what is required. Examinations reinforce the focus on disease, and ignore the importance of the patient as a psycho-social being (Kurtz et al. 1985). The experiments at McMaster and Harvard Universities are limited, since those students must take the same licensing exams as do graduates from more traditional medical schools, and as yet there is no evidence to suggest that the McMaster-trained physician is different from graduates of other schools.

Sociologists acknowledge that medical education plays a limited role in the socialization of the physician. To understand doctoring it is necessary to be aware of the social class background, gender and ethnic composition of the profession. The predominantly male, upper-middle class, white/anglo background of physicians in Canada determines to a great extent the values and beliefs of the medical profession. Medical education does not completely re-socialize individuals; it only reinforces a particular world view of an elite subculture. In addition, medicine tends to attract individuals who have an affinity for science, rather than those with superior social skills. The development of a medical practitioner is influenced not only by societal expectations of physicians but also by the student's expectations as to what it will be like to be a physician. The ideals of doctoring (to prevent suffering and heal the sick) which are part of the individual's desire to become a physician, may be quite different from the reality (Zimbardo 1972). Becoming a doctor has traditionally guaranteed the rewards of wealth, power and prestige, but this promise is being eroded by the economic and social realities of modern medical practice. Medical qualifications may no longer guarantee entrance to the wealthy elite.

Medical practice is being affected by (1) changes in the types of health problems, (2) the development of new technologies, (3) shifts in the demographic structure of the population, (4) the realization of the importance of psycho-social health needs, and (5) the realization that the physician's opinion is only one possible interpretation of what is good for the patient. To keep up with these transformations in medical practice, the educators of physicians must be more willing to adapt to the real, and not only the perceived, needs of the population.

Summary

This chapter discusses the growing complexity of the health-care industry in Canada. It also discusses the control of the medical profession over medical practice and how this control is declining as provincial governments take over the definitions of health and health care. The traditional medical control over medical treatment has been supported by medical education, ways of transmitting information, historical precedent and the social relations between physician and patient.

Physicians and nurses, as health-care professionals, are taking on more complex roles and authority in society and in health care. Although nurses are being given more responsibility, their status as a profession independent of medicine is doubtful. The class, gender and ethnic backgrounds of physicians are important factors in the relation between physicians and other health-care workers, and between physicians and the public.

One of the major aims of this chapter was to start questioning the physician's ability to make decisions about the health of individuals and of the population. It is difficult to understand in whose interests decisions are made, when physicians are influenced by their authority, income and place in the social structure.

Notes

1. Many sociologists argue that the process of specialization in society is causing alienation, as individuals lose any understanding of the purpose of the whole.
2. The historical basis for this approach is in the development of scientific management, which equates efficiency and productivity with profits.
3. Approximately half of all female nurses work part time (Canada 1978 and 1983g). Nursing, as part-time work, is decreasing since women can get better pay working in the service sector, for example at supermarket check-outs.
4. There are some anomalies in this regard. In many provinces there are nurses who practise in isolated northern communities. In this situation they are given some of the powers usually reserved for doctors, since doctors are in short supply. However, when these nurses return to the more populated areas where there are doctors, they are no longer permitted to do these tasks. In many cases when nurses attempt to take over the tasks of physicians, they are prohibited from doing so. Other examples of nurses performing tasks usually reserved for doctors are midwives and nurse practitioners.
5. Many physicians disagree with this and say that there is no "doctor glut" (Ryten and Watanabe 1987).
6. The restricting of billing numbers does not prohibit physicians from setting up a practice. It simply means that they will not be able to bill the provincial government for their work, but instead have to collect a fee from each patient.
7. There is some evidence from the U.S. that a slowdown or strike by physicians actually increases the general health of the population because there is less elective surgery (Roemer and Schwartz 1979; Roemer 1981). It would be useful to find out if the Ontario doctors' strike had the same consequences.
8. When nurses or hospital workers strike there is considerable pressure put upon them by the government and the public. Many of them are charged with offenses and jailed; however, physicians are not punished for striking.
9. Nurses I have talked to say that often the woman's doctor is not present at the birth and the child is delivered by the nursing staff. This happens especially on weekends.
10. The information on physicians' incomes can be confusing because of the different terms used. There is *gross income* (the total amount

earned), *taxable income* (gross income minus the allowable deductions for running a business) and *net* or *after-tax income*. Since physicians are independent businessmen and women, not on salary as your professor is, they can reduce their taxable income by deducting expenses incurred to run their business. For example, a physician can deduct the cost of his books, but a professor cannot. In addition, because of the large income a physician can command, more disposable income is left after expenses, and this can be used to reduce tax payments through investment; many of the advertisements in physicians' magazines are for investment ventures.

11. This redevelopment of private practice in Britain is causing many problems since the government is refusing to put money into the public health system. If a patient wants immediate special care she must see a physician privately; however, that physician is using the institutions and equipment of the public health system to treat his patient. There is in effect a two-tier system, which leaves those who cannot afford the private costs to sit and wait for needed medical attention.

12. There is also a conflict between the nurses' experience of their education and of their subsequent work, and the vision they had before entering nursing school.

13. An article in the *Winnipeg Free Press*, 23 July 1986, reported an increase in drug addiction among nurses, which was attributed to stress and isolation on the job.

14. However, there is increasing pressure on physicians to join their provincial medical associations.

15. The works of Hamowy (1984) and Naylor (1986) are excellent sources on the politics involved in the control of licensing and health insurance.

16. There are many examples of physicians abusing their position of power. For example, the Ontario Medical Association acknowledged that 12 to 14 percent of physicians will have or have had drug-related problems. This is blamed on their easy access to drugs (*Winnipeg Free Press*, 27 October 1983).

17. Abraham Flexner was commissioned by the Carnegie Foundation to report on medical education in North America. His report, which was instrumental in setting the guidelines for current medical education in the U.S. and Canada, proposed a model of education based on science (biology and chemistry) and clinical practice. Johns Hopkins medical school was used as the model for his proposals.

18. Although Canada and the United States have different medical systems, medical education in Canada is influenced by that in the United States, including its ideology and focus. This may account for the fact that Canadian doctors see themselves as businessmen.

Chapter 6

Institutional and Alternate Care

The Development of Hospitals

Illness creates a group of individuals who are dependent upon other members of their community. Some societies develop elaborate social and family networks for treating illness, and others develop special institutions. Within Western culture, the hospital or **hospice** developed early on to provide social assistance to the family or to care for travellers, the sick, the poor, the insane and the old. Hospitals have historically played the role of caring for those the family or community refused to help; the psychiatric hospital is a typical example. However, these early institutions offered little treatment.

Only recently, during the 20th century, have hospitals become the primary institutions for health care. Hospitals in Canada have grown to be not only places for care and treatment but also places for rehabilitation, education, training and research (Coe 1978, 297).

Many historians state that there was a smooth evolution of the hospital from its historical beginnings as a small hospice to the large, technologically advanced institution. This gradual development is said to have been accomplished through bureaucratic re-organization for greater efficiency, and the integration of new medical discoveries into regular hospital practice. This view of hospital development uses an evolutionary model.

An alternative, developmental model states that hospitals appeared with other institutions as a response to the development of capitalism. The hospital movement in 19th-century Canada was started by "religious orders, groups of prominent citizens (non-profit lay corporations), or by municipalities . . . general hospitals were often merely places of shelter for the chronically ill poor, while the rich and the middle classes received care at home or at the doctor's office" (Torrance 1987, 480). Torrance goes on to illustrate that the development of the 20th-century Canadian hospital with its advanced division of labour, increased centralization of facilities and reliance on medical technology, was a product of its times, not isolated from societal changes.

The evolutionary perspective fails to consider the problems created by the centralized organization of health care in hospitals. It also fails to deal with the question of whether or not mortality rates were higher in hospitals than outside because of their poor condition or because hospitals are places of death.[1] The rise of iatrogenic illnesses and nosocomial infections forces us to look critically at hospital development. The assumption that hospitals became beneficial only after science became the mode of practice has been severely criticized in recent years (McKeown 1979; Hamilton 1987). These studies document the fact that hospital care is closely linked to the health and illness of the general population. There is a critical acknowledgement of problems connected with hospital treatment and a realization that institutions create as well as solve problems, while reflecting general population and societal trends.

Sanazaro (1971), using a developmental model, suggests that even though hospitals were the "crossroads of the science, art, politics, and economics of medicine, [they had] no functions independent of the advancing health services for people" (Sanazaro 1971, 132). In the 19th century hospitals developed independently of each other and were subject to their benefactors, who were either the community or physicians. The numbers of hospitals and the number of beds per 1000 population were the measure of the level of health services. At the beginning of the 20th century there was a change in the role of the hospital; it began to respond to community needs. Even though the hospital is now the central institution of health-care services, and until recently beds were a measure of services, the movement for the improvement of health-care services in the future must take place outside the hospital. Although the hospital today is the organizer of health services, it is increasingly becoming only a component within the larger system of health services (Sanazaro 1971, 138).

The Hospital in the Twentieth Century

The Hospital as Factory

Since the early 20th century, hospitals have become the focal point of health service in Canada. They are also the largest employer of health-care workers. There are over 1,200 hospitals in Canada, employing approximately 476,000 full-time and part-time workers. "This represents a bigger part of the labour force than that employed in many primary and secondary industries – for instance, more than are employed in auto manufacturing, iron and steel mills and pulp and paper mills combined (Torrance 1987, 476). Hospitals have grown to such an extent that they have been referred to as "health factories" (Friedson 1966-67; Torrance 1987). The number and costs of hospitals are increasing along with the specialization of hospital type. However, beds and patient days per 1000 population are decreasing, and many Canadians see this change as a reduction in health services.

FIGURE 6.1

PATIENT DAYS BY MAJOR CAUSES, GENERAL AND ALLIED HOSPITALS, BY SEX, CANADA, 1980-81

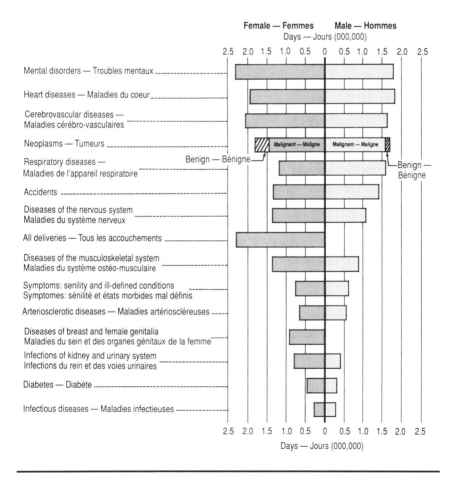

SOURCE: *Hospital Morbidity: 1979-80 and 1980-81.* Ottawa: Statistics Canada, 1984. P. 17. Catalogue 82-206. Reproduced with permission of the Minister of Supply and Services Canada.

Some of the advantages of the centralization of health services in 20th-century hospitals are: (1) the close proximity of medical knowledge and technology to the patient; (2) the efficiency and immediacy of treatment to the injured; (3) the close relationship between teaching, research and patient care facilities; and (4) the segregation of potentially harmful diseases. Disadvantages to this trend to centralization are: (1) the location of health care in large urban centres means that rural and northern areas are left without care; (2) distances between hospital and families grow, eliminating the potential for emotional and familial support to the patient; (3) the size of hospitals necessitates bureaucratic organization and has an alienating effect on the patient; and (4) since hospitals are the centre for diseases, there is a greater chance of contracting a disease while in a hospital. The tendency in Canada toward urbanization, greater centralization and specialization of health-care facilities, and the organization of hospitals as factories is increasing. This heightens the advantages and disadvantages described above.

In 1980-1981, Canadians used 48 million hospital patient days. (See Figure 6.1, above.) It is important to analyze the use of hospitals for certain types of illnesses in order to get a picture of those treated in hospitals. There are many individuals in general hospitals who should not be there, and who might be better cared for in a specialty or community institution, which would be decentralized and less expensive. Community psychiatric institutions in Saskatchewan, Health Service Organizations in Ontario and Birthing Hospitals in England are examples of decentralized health-care. Other alternatives to hospitals are discussed later in this chapter.

Health-care costs in general, and hospital costs in particular, are on the rise. This rise in costs is a major factor in the search for alternate forms of care. The Economic Council of Canada states that hospital costs accounted for 40% of the increase in health spending from 1960 to 1980. "In Canada, hospitals of all types (general and allied special, mental, and federal) made up 41.4 percent of total health care spending in 1982" (Evans 1984, 160). A significant question for those working in health-care planning is whether the dramatic rise in the costs of patient care has any effect on the health of the population (Evans 1984, 164). The answer is hard to determine for Canada as a whole, since hospitals are a provincial responsibility and there are great differences in policies and services offered across Canada. "For instance, the rate of hospital admissions for each thousand in population was 17 per cent below the national average in Quebec and 38 per cent above the national average in Saskatchewan" (Silversides 1987b). Table 6.1 gives a picture of hospital utilization in Canada.

TABLE 6.1
HOSPITAL BED CAPACITY AND UTILIZATION, CANADA, 1946-1982/83

	Public General Hospitals				Public Allied Special Hospitals		All Hospitals	
	Beds per 1000 Pop'n	Patient-Days per 1000 Pop'n	Expenditure per patient-day $current	$1971	Beds per 1000 Pop'n	Patient-days per 1000 Pop'n	Beds per 1000 Pop'n	Patient-days per 1000 Pop'n
1946	3.87	1101.4	5.27	11.72	0.45	104.8	10.13	–
1951	4.19	1212.1	9.05	13.72	0.71	201.2	10.42	–
1956	4.67	1350.2	15.95	23.28	0.66	195.4	10.84	3202.3
1961	4.86	1434.4	24.34	32.47	0.65	205.1	10.58	3368.4
1966	5.27	1527.7	38.56	46.18	0.84	266.5	10.35	3261.4
1971	5.49	1595.9	66.61	66.61	0.92	300.8	9.78	3002.0
1975	5.66	1554.0	121.82	87.93	1.02	333.7	9.18	2675.7
1976	5.15	1435.0	140.13	94.13	1.55	500.9	7.19	2062.4
1977/78	5.25	1478.1	151.87	94.45	1.57	506.8	7.14	2075.1
1978/79	5.19	1472.9	166.26	94.90	1.57	515.9	7.10	2081.9
1979/80	5.11	1438.6	182.18	95.27	1.57	523.0	6.97	2079.2
1980/81	5.11	1474.8	208.89	99.20	–	513.5*	6.98	2039.4*
1981/82	–	1471.4	236.75	99.94	–	501.8*	–	2030.2*
1982/83	5.04	1464.2	276.67	105.40	1.51	493.4	6.82	2028.8

SOURCE: R.G. Evans, *Strained Mercy: The Economics of Canadian Health Care*. Toronto: Butterworths, 1984. P. 162.

*These data are drawn from preliminary annual reports, which in earlier years are inconsistent with the subsequently published annual reports.

Most Canadian hospitals are not-for-profit institutions, and are owned by their provinces, municipalities, religious orders or voluntary organizations. The typical hospital is run by a board of directors composed of community members, administrators and physicians. Since the late 19th century, our modern hospitals, as large organizations, have taken on a model similar to other organizations; they have operated on the basis of making a profit.

In public hospitals, the goal is not profits but economic efficiency which will, it is claimed, cut costs in times of financial crisis. The move is toward "privatization." This means that previously government-owned and administered companies or institutions are sold to the private sector. The assumption is that this change will be more efficient or at least lose less money. In Canada the total privatization of the health-care system is not possible; however, there is a growing belief that hospitals are in need of better economic management. This movement toward efficiency in hospital functioning pits health considerations against efficiency, or more correctly the decisions of physicians against the decisions of administrators.

Authority Conflicts Within the Hospital

Denton (1978) states that within the organizational structure of the hospital there are three separate groupings, each with different goals. These are the occupational, administrative and authority groupings. Within each hospital, individuals are divided into different groups with opposing interests, for example doctors and nurses, administrators and medical personnel, and labour and management. This organizational complexity within the hospital is referred to by many authors as a dual line of authority. Its effect is to pit medical considerations against management considerations (Cockerham 1986, 211-17).

Cockerham sees the hospital as both a bureaucracy or formal organization, and as the professional domain of physicians. He argues that the two sides are not necessarily compatible because the professional is expected to make autonomous judgements about a patient's health, while the administrator makes judgements which are fixed by the rules and regulations of the institution. For example, physicians will usually use every means available to save a life, while administrators will point out that all means are not available, or if they are, they are not available for everyone. As a consequence, a decentralized system of authority has developed which may confuse those who, like nurses, are responsible to the physicians' orders and at the same time to hospital administrators' orders. The outcome of this separation of powers in the hospital and the fact that doctors are legally responsible to the hospital leads to attempts by administrators to take greater control over hospital physicians.

Mechanic (1978) says that the organizational problems which arise in the hospital are brought about by the costs of providing care. Physicians and administrators may come into conflict over the amount of resources to be utilized in the treatment of patients. This leads to the rationalization of care (that is, setting a standard of care for all which is applied in every situation) and an accountability by the physician for treatment and use of hospital resources.

The dual line of authority in the hospital is made more complex by the horizontal division of labour. Denton (1978) notes that the proliferation of hospital facilities and medical and administration specialties has made the hospital more complex and difficult to administer and coordinate. In response to this, many hospitals attempt to impose strict rules on all workers in the hospital. The greater the number of rules and regulations within the hospital, the greater the potential for physicians to lose control over diagnosis and treatment, and the greater the potential for the proletarianization of physicians.

The lines of authority, professional and bureaucratic, will continue to be a problem area in hospital organization, since physicians and administrators approach the problem of hospital care from different perspectives. There will continue to be conflicts as to who has the ultimate control of hospital care.

Hospital Authority and the Patient

Once admitted to the hospital, the patient is subject to its rules and regulations, either formal or informal. The patient "is faced with many restrictions on his behaviour and many directions about how he should or should not act that he did not have to observe outside the institution" (Roth 1985, 247). Even though hospital services are oriented to the notion of the welfare of patients, treatment must take place within an orderly and rational atmosphere where everyone acts appropriately. Patients usually learn the rules of the hospital through observation or being told not to do a certain thing.

Hospital personnel are subject to rules about their performance as professionals, and patients are categorized by illness and expected to obey hospital routine. Patients, therefore, are not part of the authority structure of the hospital. They have little control over their lives in hospital and are told to follow the staff's orders.[2] It could be argued that this situation is necessary in order for a hospital to run efficiently; however, it strips the patient of her identity and she loses control over her life while in the hospital. With efficiency and standardization comes depersonalization.

In a Manitoba study of more than 10,000 separate decisions about a patient's treatment, Degner and Beaton (in York 1987) found that in 90% of the cases, patients had no control over treatment decisions. Even when patients wanted to have some input, they found it very difficult. "Patients and their families have almost no control over the treatment decisions made by hospital staff during life-threatening illnesses" (York 1987).

The process of depersonalization influences the self-concept of the patient and places stress on the staff as well. The removal of the patient's identity, social support and the transformation of her daily routine only adds to the isolation felt in surrendering one's body to others. Isolation and depersonalization increase with the severity of treatment and increased use of technology. For example, in the intensive care unit (ICU) the patient is hooked up to a mechanical ventilator which helps her breathe. Because of the complex technology used in these units and the necessary restraint of the patient, isolation and loss of self become extreme (Hudelson 1977).

Upon entering the hospital the patient surrenders her personal identity, her control over resources, and responsibility for her life. This surrender is part of the process of conformity to hospital rules and regulations. From the perspective of hospital workers, patients need to be cared for; they are sick and want to be taken care of and get better.[3] By giving up the right to make decisions about their lives, patients empower physicians and nurses to make decisions about what is "good" for them. Patients who follow the routine and orders are labelled as "good." Those who ask too many questions or do not follow the routine are labelled as "bad."[4]

Hospitals and Technology

Cockerham (1986, 203) states that there are three major factors in the development of 20th-century hospitals as places where patients of all social classes ". . . could reasonably expect to be cured of their disorders." These factors are linked with the introduction of medical technology in the hospital setting. First, hospitals became centres of scientific medicine where physiology and anatomy were devoutly encouraged. Also, discoveries in bacteriology and anesthesiology allowed surgery to be developed with less pain and threat to the patient's health. Second, hospitals developed various antiseptic measures to eliminate infection and assist in the development of medical technology, for example, masks, gloves and sterilized medical instruments. Third, hospital personnel were improved; nurses and technicians were given special training in the use of new technologies and taught to assist physicians in the hospital care of patients. Finally, because of the great costs involved, the centralization of technology in hospitals made it available to all physicians and their patients. Thus, hospitals are becoming more specialized over time and their accessibility to all Canadians is limited by geography.

Technology: More Is Better?

"For most sectors of the economy, new technologies that are adopted and used are assumed to improve the efficiency or the quality of production" (Sisk, Behney and Banta 1984, 10). These innovations are assumed to reduce labour costs and save on long-term costs. In the case of medicine and health care, many new diagnostic technologies are said to reduce the costs of hospitalization through efficiency and better diagnosis.[5]

Within our culture there is an idea that the more technology we use, the better our health will be. This view is not supported by the evidence on the increased use of technology within medical practice. Even though "early studies assumed more services were synonymous with better quality care" (Sisk, Behney and Banta 1984, 11) many of the common and costly procedures now routinely administered have not been proven beneficial to health or medical costs. In fact, many of the new technologies introduced into hospitals actually cause problems and increase costs because the staff must be retrained to use them (Mumford 1983, 371).

The manner in which medicine is funded in Canada only encourages the increased use of medical technology without consideration for its economic or health benefits. Physicians are paid more to use more complex technology. There is much discussion within provincial governments about the high demand for new technologies by physicians. The demand is always for the latest equipment available, which is very expensive. Recently there have been questions about the efficacy of this new technology. Specifically, governments have asked why technology is simply an "add on" and does not replace older technology. (For example, CT scanners do not replace x-ray machines.) Further, they have pointed out that new technology creates an unlimited demand for even more. New technologies in health care are introduced and routinely used without appropriate caution for costs or possible technology-induced illness. Patients are often used as guinea pigs.

There are many examples of the inappropriate use of diagnostic services and technology. For example, in 1980 x-rays cost Canadians $275 million a year while laboratories cost $350 million a year to operate. There are considerable differences in technology use among provinces, but no noticeable difference in diagnostic ability or health levels. "Among the provinces, the number of x-rays per patient varies by more than 150 per cent, and the use of laboratory units per patients by 131 per cent" (Bennett and Krasney 1980, 63).

Today, physicians and hospitals are constantly asking their provincial governments for more funds to keep medicine up to date with the latest technology, in order to provide Canadians with the best medical care available. They argue that, while technology is initially expensive, it will save money in the long run. However, most new technology is out of date in five years. In some cases the technology has replaced workers and therefore increased efficiency and reduced costs. However, this has not been true for all new technologies.

Analysts and clinicians concerned with developing more scientifically based information on the indication for use of technologies have pointed out that technologies such as the CT scanner, elective hysterectomy, tonsillectomy, breast cancer surgery, common forms of diagnosis X-ray, and electronic fetal monitoring are being used without adequate information on their efficacy, safety, and costs. (Sisk, Behney and Banta 1984, 13)[6]

Some experts see technology as unnecessary and harmful. Dubos (1959) shows that humanitarian and social reform did much to increase the health of the population without laboratory medicine and modern diagnostic procedures. Illich (1976) goes further by pointing out that the increase in the use of modern diagnostic equipment actually produces illness.

There is still pressure by physicians to have more and better technology to treat their patients. The idea that "more equals better" permeates our society. In a 1978 Harris Poll (Harris et al. 1978) 71% of the population of the United States and 49% of physicians answered yes to the question: "Does more money equal more health?" Yet the assumption that more money and technology will increase the health of the population and save lives is contradicted by the evidence. The best possible treatment is not necessarily the most expensive.

Technology and Diagnosis

Medical technology has been used extensively in the field of diagnosis. Physicians no longer have to rely on their own judgement or on qualitative information, but can use the appropriate test or procedure to come up with "hard facts" about what is wrong with the specific part of the patient's body. Yet the procedure may be harmful to the individual (x-rays are an example) while offering only limited information. The routine use of such procedures ignores their potential dangers (Laws 1977).

Reliance on technology in diagnosis goes with the assumption that the information provided by non-human sources is unbiased and flawless. Physicians implicitly argue that such information will increase their ability to help their patients. However, this is not the case. Not only do physicians still have to interpret the test findings, they have to be familiar enough with recent advances in technology to order the correct tests for the illness in question.

It is difficult to estimate the value of diagnostic technology. The CT scanner, for example, provides raw data on the evidence of a suspected disease. These data must be analyzed in light of the patient's condition and to the extent of the physician's or technologist's ability to interpret the information (Esser and Johnston 1984). In theory, the CT is used to look for something suspected by the physician. However, it could be used in a case where the physician does not know what is wrong with the patient, and is looking for some clue that would lead to a diagnosis.

Zola (1972) states that the increased use of technology does not increase the physician's mastery over illness but does increase his authority over his patients. The care of the patient is no longer foremost in his mind; his concern is knowledge about the particular disease.

Many researchers (Cochrane 1972) challenge the usefulness of information provided by modern diagnostic equipment. One routine procedure which has been harshly criticized is cardiac catheterization. This procedure is used to find out if a patient is having problems with her heart muscle (cardiomyopathy). The test cost $350 in 1976 and resulted in the death of one out of every fifty patients. No evidence shows that it extends the life or comfort of the patient (Illich 1976, 102).

Another procedure in standard use in Canadian hospitals is foetal monitoring (Evans 1984, 227-28). Its purpose is to monitor the **foetus** and detect any distress which may call for intervention by caesarean section. However, this procedure has been shown to do more harm than good (Banta and Thacker 1979) and has initiated an epidemic of caesarean sections in the past ten years (Evans 1984, 227).

Many other new technologies which have become part and parcel of standard operating procedure, such as Critical Care Units and Intensive Care Units, have yet to prove their efficacy.

When it comes to diagnosing the cause of death, technology has not superseded traditional methods. Autopsies remain the final way to confirm or negate the physician's diagnosis. (An autopsy is a postmortem examination of a body to determine the cause of death.) Unfortunately, the rate of autopsies is declining (Smith 1984; Price and McCormick 1981). Some evidence from spot checks shows that in 40% of cases, the cause of death is incorrectly diagnosed.

> In a study of 100 consecutive cases of autopsy-proved heart attacks . . . the correct diagnosis of heart attack had been made in just 53 per cent of the cases. This compared to figures of 65 percent in 1938, 57 percent in 1948, 69 percent in 1957, and 61 percent in 1959 . . . Surprisingly, these figures came from times when blood and other diagnostic tests for heart attacks were considered less precise than they are now. (*American Funeral Director* 1984)

Not only is diagnostic ability declining with the increase in medical technology (*American Funeral Director* 1984), there is also pressure on physicians not to do autopsies that would show the ineffectiveness of the new technologies and the decline in the abilities of pathologists (Smith 1984).

To sum up this section on technology, medical practice is moving toward greater use of technology not only because of the belief that it will increase the health of the population, but also because of the demand for more exact information on a patient's condition.[7] Medical administrators, either government, hospital or clinic, firmly believe in the economic efficiency of medical technology. Physicians, since their role is saving lives and improving patient health, usually have little concern for the costs of care.

Medicine is no longer the art that it once was, and diagnosis and treatment are now relegated to formulae which link the patient to technology and subvert the role of the physician. Also, medical technology has a tendency to create more costs than it eliminates (Deber and Leatt 1986). These new diagnostic technologies are probably more profitable for those who manufacture and use them, than for patients who are subjected to them (Evans 1984, 276).

Other considerations in trying to understand the role of medical technology in the health of Canadians are: (1) the manufacture and development of medical technologies by corporations whose goals are not health but profits; (2) the quality of life of individuals affected by technology; (3) the experimental nature of some techniques; and (4) the transformation of the sick individual into an object through the increase in the use of medical technology.

Finally, technology supports the general trend to objectifying the patient. Technology further separates doctors from patients and focuses the goal of medical practice on the disease rather than on the patient's health. The total reliance on the medical model has a tendency to push physicians to accept new techniques of medical investigation, leaving the real world of the patient behind.

The Costs of Hospital Care

There is great pressure to change our current system of health care, largely because of how much this system is costing. Many say that there is a health-care crisis in Canada and that this crisis is the result of a health-cost crisis. Why is health care becoming so costly and how can the situation be changed?

In 1960 health-care expenditures were just over $2 billion and in 1982 they were $30 billion, a fifteen-fold increase (Canada 1983f, 4). However, if we take into consideration inflation and the percentage of our Gross Domestic Product (GDP) spent on health care, the situation looks different. For example, in constant dollars (1971), which take account of inflation, the per capita (per person) costs rose from $165 to $445, an increase of less than three times. Health costs as a percentage of our GDP rose from 5.6% in 1960 to 7.3% in 1970 and to 8.4% in 1982 (Canada 1983f, 8). Comparison of health costs between countries can give a relative mark to our spending. While Canada's costs are higher than in Britain (which has a more socialized system), they are lower than in the U.S. (which has a more private system).

Therefore, while actual costs of health care are increasing, they have been held down over the past 25 years by provincial and federal government intervention. It could be argued that the crisis in health-care financing would be much worse if federal and provincial governments had not intervened. Two major government responses to the concern with health expenditures have been the Lalonde Report (1974), which argued that individuals should be more responsible for their own health, and the Established Programs Financing Act (1977), which started transferring more health-care costs from the federal to the provincial government. Since the 1984 election of the Conservative government in Canada, and the subsequent election of many provincial Conservative governments, there has been a movement toward the privatization of public agencies, health care included (Soderstrom 1982).

The areas of greatest health expenditure in Canada are hospitals and physicians (Blomquist 1979, 125). In 1982, hospitals and various health-care homes used 53.7% of health-care expenditures, and payments to physicians used 14.7% (Canada 1983f, 10). Hospital operating costs in Canada have increased dramatically. They accounted for 40% of the increase in health-care spending between 1960 and 1980 (Silversides 1987c). Between 1947 and 1982 hospital spending went from 1.27% of GDP to 3.5% (Evans 1984, 9).

Since hospital care is labour-intensive, the greatest cost of hospital care is wages. In 1977, 70% of hospital operating costs were fees, salaries and wages (Stektasa 1977, 5). From 1967 to 1977, 3/4 of the increase in hospital costs can be accounted for by 12% per year increase in fees, wages and salaries.

Cost increases in hospitals can be traced to other sources, besides wages. The increased use of technology is an important factor, as shown in the preceding pages. Allentuck (1978) found that between 1970 and 1974 laboratory work increased 52.7% and diagnostic radiology 22%, yet the hospital mortality rate did not decrease significantly. One explanation for this increased number of tests is the increase in physicians and their increased use of tests. The previous chapter showed how the increase of physicians and their workloads generates more demand for medical care and increases the overall costs of health care (Evans 1973, 164). The rise in the cost of hospital care can also be attributed to the increased use of expertise, labour and drugs. Inputs to treatment in hospitals grew at an annual average of 6.2% between 1965 and 1975. However, labour costs grew only 0.6% per year for the same period, while medical supplies grew 4.0% (Bennett and Krasney 1980).

Of course, costs also increase with the severity of the patient's accident or illness. Acute illnesses are the most costly, and care in acute-care hospitals is the most expensive. In 1977 acute-care hospital costs were five times those of home care and three times those of chronic institutional care (Bennett and Krasney 1980). Among Western countries, Canada has one of the highest rates of hospital treatment, length of stay in hospital, and numbers of the population who are treated in hospital. These rates may be attributed to the history of health care in Canada: hospitals were the first part of the health-care system to be subsidized by the government. "The rising costs of health care are simply the price we pay for adhering to the ideal that every sick person is entitled to the best possible treatment" (Blomquist 1979, 5). One solution to the cost crisis in health care is to reduce acute hospital care. However, this solution should not be forced on individuals or communities where there is little organized care and where there is a great possibility of social hardship, especially where chronic care has to be paid for.

Dramatic changes are taking place in Canadian society. The population structure is changing, the major causes of death are changing, the types and costs of technology are changing,[8] the structure of the medical profession is changing, and the methods of funding health-care costs are changing. Many argue that we need a new paradigm or way of thinking to address these concerns. Any new paradigm, however, will threaten the established guardians of health care and those of the population who cling to the medical model.

Alternatives to Hospital Care

Our current universal health-care system in Canada, which we now all assume as a given, was bitterly opposed by the medical profession at the time of its inception. It was a radical departure from the private health-care system traditionally practised in Canada before the 1960s (Badgley and Wolfe 1967). The progressive movement for a universal health-care system, which does not make distinctions on the basis of wealth, grew out of the economic and political thrust of the post-World War II cooperative movement (CCF) which developed in Saskatchewan.

Alternatives to the hospital are today being sought because of our current economic situation and the political will of Canadians for the right to health care, and again these alternatives are being opposed by physicians. These developments, along with the reduction in federal transfer payments[9], are forcing provincial governments to restructure their methods of providing health care and to look for innovative, less costly alternatives to hospital care.[10]

Many of the problems associated with the development of new forms of care can be traced to the conflict between physicians and provincial government administrators. The issue is who is to define care and how it is to be administered.[11]

Because of current legislation, the provinces are forced into models of alternate care which do not shift the costs to patients.[12] The increase in numbers and types of care alternatives available to the population gives more power to the provincial governments, which are the final consumers of services. For the medical profession, it would be more advantageous to keep the costs of payment in the hands of the mass of patients, who are more disorganized. For example, a Nova Scotia physician argues: "What's forgotten here is the responsibility of the user ... The government is against a user fee. I call it a responsibility fee" (Moulton 1987, 30). A question we should ask is: who should be responsible to whom (individual to physician, or physician to government) and who should be controlled by whom? Much of the discussion about alternate care funding centres on physician control.

Many alternatives to hospital care are developing. Alternatives to acute hospital care include Community Clinics, Health Service Organizations and various day-surgery and alternate care clinics. Alternatives to chronic care in hospital are the hospice or chronic care hospital. There are also private, physician-controlled alternatives to hospital care: the group physician clinic and the shopping mall practice. Since each province is free to choose the direction its health-care system will take, it is likely that different alternatives will develop in different provinces.

Community Clinics and Health Service Organizations

The Clinic or Health Service Organization (HSO) is an alternative to the acute-care hospital. These organizations are not physician-controlled, but are under community guidance. Community Clinics originated in Saskatchewan, as did much of the present-day Canadian health-care system (Wolfe 1964). Since the province has a history of cooperative institutions and progressive health care, it was logical that the general ideology of the cooperative movement be incorporated in its hospital system. Other provinces have since followed Saskatchewan's lead: for example, HSOs (Michaels 1982) and day-surgery hospitals (Pablo and Cleary 1982) have been established in Ontario. The HSOs of Ontario are group practices providing almost all types of care to their patient population (Michaels 1982). Many who work in the HSO say it is ideal since they can devote time to their patients, rather than being pressed to see as many as possible (Barr 1983, 253). Also, within the HSO or the clinic, non-medical (and therefore less costly) personnel can be used to assist in patient care. However, physicians outside the HSOs argue that they offer no incentive for better care, as does the fee-for-service system. They also argue that doctors are told by the institution's administrators what kind of treatment they can give their patients, and non-physician care is viewed as inferior. The development of health-care services along the line of the HSOs fits the model of the proletarianization of physicians, discussed in the last chapter, by reducing their power and independence.

Paying the Physicians

They [clinics] serve a defined population group of enrollees, and their revenues are a fixed dollar amount per enrollee per time period. Enrollees are then provided with all "needed" services, as judged by the group's practitioners, either from the group itself or from external referrals at the group's expense. (Evans 1984, 149)

These clinics use either a capitation system or a global budget system. Under the capitation system, the clinic receives a monthly payment from government for each patient enrolled in the clinic; the physicians in the clinic are usually paid a set fee for each patient they see, no matter what treatment is given. In the global budget system, the clinic is paid a lump sum for all its services, no matter how many times a patient needs care, and the physicians are paid a salary. In both these systems, all services needed are provided by the clinic. Capitation has been recommended for the new HSO in Manitoba and is practised in Ontario HSOs and Saskatchewan Clinics.

Problems and Conflicts

There are some problems and conflicts in connection with the introduction of group health clinics. One is the relationship between members of the staff: specifically, how the different specialties are paid (Ghan and Road 1971) and how the medical staff relates to the non-medical staff (Light and Kleiber 1978). There are also conflicts between clinic physicians and lay boards of directors over policies, staffing, payment and goals of the clinic. Arguments over who has the right and responsibility to focus the goals of the clinic pit the community's interests against the doctors'.

Community-Minded Physicians

As may be apparent by now, HSOs and Clinics attract a certain type of doctor. Physicians who decide to work in clinics are those who are willing to make less money and put community interests ahead of their own.[13] They are also willing to work with the general community in setting health goals (Mahood 1973). However, many physicians are *not* willing to participate in such clinics (partly because of the ideas of medical practice put forward in medical schools) and are not willing to be accountable to non-medical administrators.

Do Clinics Cut Costs?

An issue of much debate is whether the HSO or Community Clinic reduces health-care costs by keeping people out of the hospital. Some argue that clinics do reduce the costs of health care by reducing the amount and length of hospital care used by their enrollees (McPhee 1974; Evans 1984, 149-50). Others, arguing from the medical profession's perspective (Baltzan 1973; Brandejs 1973), state that clinics do not decrease the rates of hospitalization and thus do not decrease the costs of health care. However, recent information from the United States shows a significant drop in hospitalization by the users of HSOs (called HMOs in the U.S.).

Alternate Care for the Elderly and Chronically Ill

Hospital care is not only costly. Many patients, such as the chronically ill elderly, do not need to be in a hospital and would rather not be there. In Canada, 6.7% of individuals over 65 and 33% of those over 85 are in nursing homes and other institutions for the chronically ill and elderly (Chappell et al. 1986, 81). Most of the chronically ill come from the elderly portion of our population, and those over 64 use more hospital services than those who are younger (McDaniel 1986, 81-82). Table 6.2 indicates the extent of hospital use by those under and over 65 years.

TABLE 6.2

SHORT-TERM HOSPITALIZATION IN TERMS OF BED DAYS, DISCHARGES AND LENGTH OF STAY, CANADA 1978-79

	Age ≤64	Age 65+
Bed days per 1,000 population per year*	1161	5186
Discharges per 1,000 population per year	119	280
Average length of stay (days)**	9.7	18.0

SOURCE: Adapted from N. Chappell et al., *Aging and Health Care: A Social Perspective.* Toronto: W.B. Saunders. 1986. P. 106.

* Bed days refer to the total number of days spent in hospital per year.
** Average length of stay refers to the mean number of days spent in hospital per admission.

In 1976, those 65 or older made up 9% of the population, yet they used 34% of hospital patient days (Rombout 1975). "In the early 1970s, Gomers and his associates report elderly persons occupied 22 percent of acute hospital beds and 76 percent of chronic beds" (Chappell et al. 1986, 107). Increasing numbers of hospital patients are not acutely ill, but "they have chronic and degenerative disorders which will end in death" (Skelton 1982, 556).

Skelton (1982) says that there are two problems with hospital care for the chronic patient. First, health care professionals have a difficult time dealing with care and not cure: "International studies of hospital care of the dying patient have shown consistently that less time is spent and greater delay occurs in providing attention to these individuals than is the case for patients with better prognosis" (Skelton 1982, 556). Second, chronic patients would rather be at home, in familiar surroundings.

> Of more than 100 patients who were fully aware of their imminent death, almost 80% expressed a deep desire to die in their own homes. . . . Of the individuals studied, however, 68% actually died in an institutional setting. (Skelton 1982, 557)

Hospitals are not "bastions of cure" and can do little to help those with chronic diseases.

> Some 75% of all patients in our acute care hospitals will not be cured – at best they will receive symptomatic relief. Of the 25% of the patients who are more fortunate, as many as one half will probably have self-limiting disorders which, given time, will recover spontaneously. (Skelton 1982, 556)

Even though modern medicine can relieve much of the pain associated with chronic illness, pain is not the only factor in the patient's life. A holistic approach to chronic care must take account of "anxiety, lone-liness, unresolved questions, embarrassment, difficulty in changing posi-tions in bed or chair, using the toilet and many other factors" (Skelton 1982, 558). What is needed is **palliative care**.

The economic and social strain on hospitals could obviously be reduced by changes in the way we take care of our elderly and chronically ill. The two options are community care, or some other type of institu-tional care.

Community Care

Since institutional care is the most expensive, there is a tendency to place more responsibility for chronic care on the community. In Canada, however, "a national scheme covering community based care . . . does *not* exist" (Chappell et al. 1986, 89). Community care requires a commitment on the part of provincial governments to develop or maintain the com-munity social services which assist the elderly, such as meals on wheels, therapy, and recreation and rehabilitation services. Box 6.1 gives a sum-mary of recent developments in community care.

Institutional Alternatives

The institutional alternatives for chronic care include the Chronic Care Hospital (CCH), the Day Hospital (DH), the nursing home and the hospice.

The Chronic Care Hospital (CCH) is a long-term care facility and works in much the same way as other hospitals, but admits only the chronically ill. While the CCH provides medical care, it is not holistic care as described above. Ontario, for example, has 11,000 chronic care beds and a waiting time of 2.5 years (Silversides 1987b). These Ontario CCHs have different types of beds: ward, semi-private and private. A semi-private bed can cost $7,000 per year more than a ward bed, and a private bed $14,000 extra. Many say there is discrimination in this system, since it caters to those who can afford treatment and most of the elderly are poor.

Another institutional alternative is the Day Hospital (DH), which is an extended care facility. The DH originated to take care of the needs of the many elderly with psychiatric problems who do not require complete hospitalization, but it also functions to take care of the physically ill. The DH is defined "as a place where complete hospital treatment is given under medical supervision to patients who return to their homes each night" (Pablo and Cleary 1982, 176). Parkwood Day Hospital in London, Ontario is an example of this type of DH. This model of care combines the expertise of medical treatment with the emotional support of home care. However, some families are better equipped to help the chronic patient than others. We cannot expect that every family will be economically, emotionally or socially able to provide for its elderly and chronically ill

Box 6.1

DEVELOPMENTS IN COMMUNITY CARE

Provinces differ in their service provision not so much in acute care services as in long-term care services for the elderly and handicapped. There are a number of reasons for this: differences in populations and their demands and needs; differences in attitudes to providing support services other than medical care; and differences in resources available to provincial governments.

Populations in the Prairie and Maritime provinces tend to be much more stable than those of Alberta and British Columbia. In consequence, provinces like Prince Edward Island have been accustomed to accommodating their elderly residents within extended families, whereas the elderly in British Columbia often do not have these family supports available to them. In recent years, the numbers of Canadians aged sixty-five and over has begun to increase (now approximately ten percent). Although the peak of old age dependency in the community is expected to be approximately eighteen percent, it will not come until about 2010 A.D. when the postwar baby boom population begins to move into retirement.

Some provincial governments are more committed to assisting the elderly (and the handicapped) than others. They are governments which are committed to a welfare state approach; they believe that social problems must be attacked simultaneously and that there is a connection between disease and poverty, lack of education, poor housing and unemployment. Saskatchewan, Manitoba and Quebec have led the way in organizing services for those who seek help through a social entry and not solely through a medical entry into the system – that is, the client may ask social workers (rather than physicians only) to assess their needs for support. Other provinces believe that help seeking should be a matter of adopting the sick role and going through the medical gateway. This has led to differences in the development of community services across the provinces.

The legitimacy of providing professional and other paid supportive care in the community rather than in institutions was low until the mid-seventies. Nevertheless, two kinds of home care had already begun to emerge: care required to prevent hospitalization; and care required for backup to shorter hospitalization (early discharge). Hospitals, reacting to the Task Force Report [National Health and Welfare's Task Force on the Costs of Health Care (1969)] had begun to develop some (limited) outreach or ambulatory care services, with the idea being that these medical, surgical and rehabilitation day care programs were to prevent admissions to inpatient beds of those who could manage without the full expensive treatment. But still there was little money spent on those with long-term health problems, although the development of the Canada Assistance Plan (1966) had helped to ease the lot of some impaired (but not chronically sick) people.

By the mid-seventies, the proportion of elderly in the population was growing larger and the cost of hospital care was continuing to rise. It was felt that some action was needed. The opportunity came with the Established Program Financing Act, 1977, which not only moved from tied to block grants (thus freeing the provinces in their resource allocation), but also added a new grant from the federal government for extended care (nursing home care) developments.

It will take some time for the full impact of the financing changes to be felt. Meanwhile there do not seem to be sufficient institutional beds or community support services to meet demand, at least in the more affluent provinces.

SOURCE: Crichton et al. 1984, vol. 1, 91. Reprinted with the permission of the Canadian Hospital Association and Anne Crichton, Jean Lawrence and Susan Lee from *Doctors and Patients Negotiate the System of Care: Readings in the Canadian Health Care System series.* (Ottawa: Canadian Hospital Association, 1984), P. 91.

members. In fact, placing the burden of care on the family may be a way of discriminating against certain social groups. Also, many of the elderly have no family: they live alone and in poverty (Chappell et al. 1986, Chapter 5).

A third institutional alternative for the care of the elderly is the nursing home. Chappell says that less than 10% of Canada's elderly are in these homes (in Bohuslawsky 1987). Nursing homes provide limited care and are seen by many in them as death houses. Most nursing homes are supported by government funds but some are run on a for-profit basis and thus provide only a minimal amount of care.[14] Many nursing home residents complain of inactivity, loneliness, unqualified staff and lack of rehabilitation or emotional support (Bohuslawsky 1987). Nursing homes have been defined as socially useless, as ghettos for the elderly with chronic problems, and therefore receive little attention.

The last institutional alternative is the hospice. The modern hospice movement seeks to remove from hospitals those who cannot be helped by hospital care, primarily the chronically ill. Alternatives like the hospice would not only reduce the costs of care, they would also be a more rational and humane way of dealing with chronic diseases and death. A hospice attempts to provide professional care within a holistic environment of caring and support. It attempts to deal with many of the social-psychological and chronic care problems (as when a patient has cancer, or AIDS) that are ignored by medical practice (Snider 1980). For example, in Winnipeg a voluntary women's organization established Jocelyn House as an alternative place for terminally ill cancer patients. For one-quarter of the cost of treating cancer patients in hospital, this hospice provides privacy, a tranquil home atmosphere and medical help when required. It is run more like a home than a hospital. Patients are free to use the grounds and leave for day or night visits with their families. "It would be no different from living in your own home, except that you have the 24-hour supervision that gives a terminally ill cancer patient the security of knowing there is always someone there looking out for them" (*Winnipeg Free Press*, 12 August 1986). The hospice is the best answer to what many health-care providers are demanding: a holistic, humane approach to palliative care.

Mall Medicine

A growing alternative to hospital care, especially out-patient and emergency services, is being provided by small walk-in clinics in shopping malls. Since the late 1970s mall medical centres have opened across Canada. They provide quick, convenient medical service in several health specialties: physicians, dentists, optometrists and chiropractors all work in the same office. These mall clinics are located in high density areas and are open long hours and on weekends (Oglov 1985).

Although these centres are said to provide a needed service to the population – they see about 250 patients per week (Oglov 1985, 456) – they are being criticized by governments, the medical profession and other health professionals.

First, the statement that these services are necessary because people use them cannot be accepted at face value. The convenience of these mall clinics may in fact create a greater demand for services. They also appeal to patients who want instant diagnosis and immediate treatment. It is claimed that these centres reduce the costs of care to "$22 per visit, as compared to $65 to $75 at the hospital" (Oglov 1985, 456). But many who visit these centres are also referred to their physicians or hospital emergency departments. Thus, mall clinics cause an "over-servicing" of the patient. Many provincial governments argue that these centres have not increased the health of the population, but have increased the costs of servicing the population.

Second, many physicians are opposed to the mall medicine approach because it takes patients away from private-practice physicians working a normal working day. They also think that those in mall medicine are "in it for the money," and lack concern for the quality of care. It is true that these ventures are profitable, but on the other hand they service a population who may find it too costly, in time or money, to see a physician during working hours. In other words, these centres increase competition among physicians.

Third, since these mall centres are run on the same reactive model as medical practice in general, they have little responsibility to the community. For example, they do not offer their patients education or preventive medical care. Therefore mall medicine does not offer better care; it is simply another way of packaging and marketing a product.

Finally, mall clinics provide employment for physicians without a practice and patients. Beginning physicians who cannot buy or buy into[15] a practice are attracted to such centres. They offer a way to build up a clientele and experience while being paid. (It has yet to be seen if the turnover in these centres is great.) The mall clinic option is also attractive for new physicians wishing to practise in a location where they might not otherwise be able to, especially a large city. It also provides a referral clientele from other health professionals working in the centre.

Mall medicine may also be a reaction to the "over-supply" of physicians in Canada. There is evidence to suggest that the patient pool is decreasing while the services per patient are increasing (Evans, Roch and Pascoe 1986). Physicians are competing for patients while some provincial governments are attempting to limit the numbers of physicians through the control of billing numbers, the number of positions in medical schools, and the reduced immigration of foreign doctors.[16]

Alternate Care in the Near Future

New forms of providing health care are developing throughout Canada. Partially these are being forced by: (1) the economics of care, (2) the relationship between the provincial and federal governments, (3) our belief in the right to health care, and (4) the growing demand for a more holistic and humane way of dealing with illness. Weller (1977) sees the future development of health services as responding to critiques of the current health-care system by offering holistic alternatives to the narrow focus of modern medicine. There has to be a change in the way we think about health services and who provides them. There must be a change, too, in the way health providers think about what they provide. These issues are important since there are two very different paths to choose from: either the complete socialization of medical care, or a return to privatization.

The latter alternative has already been proposed by the medical profession in Quebec, with the aim of creating competition and limiting the use of medical services. A report by the Quebec Medical Association also urges user fees because of the over-use of their vast and complex system (Shalom 1987).

Summary

Hospitals are a major component of our present medical system. However, their use is costly and does not fit current health needs of the population. In the past, hospitals acted as the seat of professional power, giving the medical profession an institutional power base. Because of the place and role of the hospital in Canada today, there are two opposing forces that are attempting to direct the future development of institutional medicine: physicians, who wish to maintain their control over treatment and care, and provincial governments, who wish to reduce costs and respond to the health demands of the population. Trends toward alternate care and institutional support will proceed slowly as forces for both privatization and further socialization of the health-care system press for political support.

The main points of this chapter are: (1) hospitals are the focal point of health care in Canada; (2) hospitals are organized along the lines of factories and other bureaucratic organizations; (3) because of this organization there are conflicts between doctors and administrators within the hospital's authority structure; (4) technological developments in health care create many problems; and (5) since hospital care is costly, a number of alternatives (clinics, hospices and mall practice) are developing.

Notes

1. It can be assumed that the probability of catching a disease is higher in places where diseases are being treated. For example, mortality rates are excessively high in intensive care units.
2. It might be argued that the illness has taken precedence over the patient.
3. Patients are grouped by illness in the hospital. This makes the administration of treatment easier but it is not necessarily beneficial for the patient.
4. Often nurses say that doctors and nurses make the worst patients. When a physician becomes a patient, the role conflict is extreme because the definitions of a good patient and a good physician are in opposition.
5. In Ontario many groups argued that the introduction of CT scanners in hospitals would be profitable in the long run since they could prevent unnecessary, expensive hospitalization (Deber and Leatt 1986).
6. The authors go on to say that inadequately assessed medical procedures range as high as 80%.
7. In response to the increase in malpractice suits in the United States, many physicians are ensuring that their judgements are well supported by scientific evidence. This practice can lead to the overuse of testing, which may be harmful to the patient. It can also increase the cost of care. Finally, tests may come to dictate diagnosis instead of supplementing the physician's judgement.
8. The turn-around time for medical technology is about five years.
9. Transfer payments are the amount the federal government gives to the provinces to help pay health-care costs. The federal government used to pay 50% of these costs, but the amounts have been dropping in recent years.
10. Provincial health-care costs are increasing and close to 30% of provincial budgets are being spent on health. For example, Nova Scotia's health-care costs have increased 52.4% in the past four years (Moulton 1987, 30).

11. Ferguson (1985), a physician, argues that administrators should have some knowledge about the process they are administering, if they are to have credibility. Since physicians know more about health than anyone else, they should start to take on the responsibility of administration.

12. Under the Canada Health Act, the federal government can withhold transfer payments to provinces that force individual patients to pay any of the cost of their care.

13. Students may have heard of the Hippocratic Oath, in which the physician swears to put the health of patients above his own personal interests. However, taking this oath is optional for physicians in Canada today.

14. The exact ratio of private to public nursing homes will vary from province to province, depending on the ideology of the government in power.

15. Many retiring physicians will sell their practice – patients, files and location – to other physicians. This is like selling a clientele. Although patients are not required to see the new physician, most do, rather than search for a new doctor.

16. Woods (1983, 1171) argues that there is not a surplus of physicians, and that the move by the government to limit the physician population is aimed at reducing costs by introducing substitute health-care workers, nurses for example, who would be less expensive than physicians.

Chapter 7

Current Issues in Health and Health Care

There are many issues which cannot be addressed in this text, for lack of room. This chapter deals with some which are of more immediate concern than others. The first section of this chapter, on health care, will discuss the rights of patients in their relations with hospitals and doctors, and will go on to suggest possible alternatives to medical care in Canada. The second section will discuss two health issues on the minds of most Canadians today, AIDS and alcoholism. The latter problems will significantly alter the lives and family relationships of those persons affected. These issues are to some extent social rather than medical concerns, though they are becoming medicalized.

Health Care

In reaction to the process of medicalization discussed earlier, individuals and groups are taking a more active role in their health and health care. First, the movement for patients' rights is attempting to educate people about the role of the patient within the system of medical care. This movement is also attempting to reintroduce the concept of the human being into medical practice. Second, those disenchanted with orthodox medical practice are looking elsewhere for health care. Various alternatives have developed to fill this need, some being more successful and legitimate than others. Their worth, however, cannot be judged by the fact that they lie outside orthodox medical science.

Patients' Rights

Many organizations exist in Canada to support and promote the interests of particular groups, which may be in a minority or lack power: women, natives and children are examples of such groups. More powerful groups, such as professions and industrial workers, also have their own organizations or unions, which work for their particular interests.

169

However, until recently, patients were unrepresented as a group, since their welfare was considered to be the domain of the physician and the hospital. Today, many provincial civil liberties associations are arguing that patients also have rights which are being overlooked (Jager 1987 and Rozovsky 1980).

As shown in the previous chapter, the patient's rights in hospital are defined by the rules and regulations of that institution. The smooth running of a hospital is based on the passivity of the patient and her willingness to do what she is told (Coburn 1980, 16). In a four-year study, Degner and Beaton (in York 1987) found that patients and their families had little control over treatment decisions. Patients who wanted to refuse certain treatments had to be insistent. Many times information was withheld from patients to ensure that treatment decisions by physicians and staff would be followed. While it is true that there are patients who wish to have the medical staff make the decisions, all patients should still have the right to know what will happen to them. This includes being informed of the side effects of certain treatments, information which in many cases is withheld from patients.

Stroman (1976, 147) defines five areas of patient rights: (1) good medical care, (2) informed consent, (3) a choice of provider, (4) self-determination in medical care, and (5) privacy, confidentiality and respect. At present patients are not guaranteed these rights. In signing consent forms (which are sometimes blank) they give the hospital and doctor more or less *carte blanche*.

The Right to Good Medical Care

The Canada Health Act of 1983 stated that every Canadian has the right to medical care, and that all Canadians would be given equal access to health care. Since health is a provincial jurisdiction, the act states that each province must guarantee: universality, portability, accessibility and comprehensiveness. The provinces, then, are responsible for the way these are ensured. Any definition of "good" or "adequate" medical care is likely to be subjective. Therefore, the definition that is enforced will be either that of the province or that of the medical profession, not the patient.

The Right to Informed Consent

The right to informed consent is the right to know exactly what will or could happen to us because of a certain treatment. Informed consent is possible only when the patient knows what risks the treatment involves and what alternatives there are. In cases of emergency treatment, this is not possible. However, in most other situations, either in hospital or out, patients could be informed about their treatments, and are not. While they are not forced to consent to treatment, in various ways they are made to feel they cannot object or even ask questions. Sometimes patients are used as the focus of an experiment, or a research project where they are screened for some disease, and are not told about this. They may be given a medication and told, "Take this and we'll see what happens."[1] This withholding of information is considered normal practice by the medical profession. It is routine for physicians to take risks with their patients, since they think it their responsibility.

The Right to a Choice of Provider

We may assume that in Canada we have the right to choose who will provide us with medical care. However, this depends on where we live; for example those living in the North have little or no choice. Second, where more specialized care is needed, our choice is more limited. Third, because of the way medical care is funded, or because of prejudice on our part, we may be restricted from choosing an alternate health-care professional. It may even be illegal to use certain providers, such as **lay midwives**. Thus geography, the medical profession, the law and our personal financial situation may restrict our choice of provider.

The Right to Self-Determination

Self-determination means being part of the process of making decisions that affect our bodies and our lives. Patients willingly give up control of their bodies to the medical profession and become objects to be studied. Patients are not included in the decisions and the process of healing. The patient's family also suffers by being excluded from the process, since they have to live and interact with the patient.

This right to self-determination is being tested by individuals who are terminally ill and by families of those being kept alive by technology, when there is no hope of recovery. Their wish is for death with dignity.

The Right to Privacy, Confidentiality and Respect

The right to privacy in a hospital is hard to maintain. Being in a large ward, especially, means losing control over one's environment, with a consequent loss of self-respect. Privacy is also lost when the patient becomes the object of discussion for the interns and residents in the hospital. This objectification of the patient disregards her autonomy and feelings, and results in a sense of loss of respect. This procedure, which is routine, may in fact contribute to the patient's illness through stress.

Patients should also have the right to confidentiality. Their charts cannot be viewed by everyone and their condition should not be talked about in the halls of the hospital.

Many people have remarked that they were treated like objects or children while in hospital. Patients should have the right to be treated as persons, but many times the structure of the health-care system works against this right. The rights of patients are now a constant issue within the health-care system. However, rights will not be freely given to patients but must be demanded, either by the patient or by those working on behalf of the patient. Many who have experienced the objectification and alienation of a hospital stay now seek alternative treatment for their ills.

Alternative Medicine

"Contemporary western medicine is a valuable but incomplete approach to health. It has concentrated on disease and neglected health" (Sobel 1979, 3). Recently in Canada there has been a movement to search out alternatives to traditional medicine (McDonnell and Valverde 1985). Some of these alternatives, such as women's health clinics and chiropractors, are within the medical model, and some like massage, lie outside the parameters of modern medical practice. In reaction to the medical model of health care, which treats the patient as an object, rather than a full human being, alternatives have developed which stress the wholeness and integration of mind, body and environment. These alternatives are becoming more attractive as modern medicine is seen to be relatively ineffective for chronic and lifestyle illnesses.

Health-care alternatives are loosely based on the idea that our physical ills have more to do with the persons, community and world around us, than with our biology. "Observations in human beings and experiments with animals establish beyond doubt that health and disease are influenced by life situations that transcend the direct impact of physiochemical forces" (Dubos 1979, 43). Also, many of these alternate forms of health care stress healing rather than cure. Note that the traditional medical system also offers few cures.

Cure is the elimination of the cause of a disease which may be life-threatening; healing includes the care of the individual throughout the illness and after the cure. For example, a cure may call for the amputation of a limb; however, the patient's subsequent adjustment to life without a limb is not considered part of the cure. Healing is concerned with more than the physical illness; it deals as well with the psychological and social problems that may arise after the cure.

The holistic approach of these alternatives is based on certain assumptions about the human body: (1) our health is determined by a balanced state of well-being; (2) our bodies have the ability to heal themselves; and (3) our interactions with those around us can affect our well-being. Techniques and practices which stress the above principles are: meditation, visualization, biofeedback, massage, acupuncture and yoga. These alternatives are not meant to replace modern medicine, but to promote wellness so that illness does not develop.[2]

As in the lifestyle approach, there is an emphasis on the ability of the individual to control her own health. As stated earlier, the problem with this approach is that it "blames the victim" for her ills. The same could be said of many who practise alternative forms of health care. No matter what the philosophy behind the approach, if it focuses on the individual, without exploring the effects of the larger social structure on our health, it is blaming the individual for her own woes (Coreil and Levin 1984-85).

Others who practise health alternatives stress interaction with the environment; they refer to a human ecology in which larger social and political factors influence our health and the ability to deal with illness (Sobel 1979, 381-86). In some recent research, psychologists (Goleman 1986) have found that our health is dependent upon the meaningful relations we have with our family and friends. The interaction between personal/emotional issues and economic/political issues is also influential.[3]

This focus on the environment is not new; in the early 20th century, before the miracle drugs, there was a movement called Social Medicine, which was concerned with public health and preventive medicine (Sand 1952).

Many of us (especially physicians) are inclined to dismiss these non-traditional alternatives as mysticism or foolishness. However, many studies indicate that some of them have positive features and do work. For example, biofeedback and acupuncture are now commonly accepted as having medical uses. Meditation is thought to be the best treatment for hypertension. If some alternate forms of treatment are useless or harmful, the same can be said of routine medical techniques and drugs.

While these alternatives to traditional medicine provide a greater choice to the health-consuming public, it must be remembered that only a limited part of the population has access to them. Usually they are available only in the larger Canadian cities. Also, many are not supported by provincial funding since they are not considered medical. Only individuals who are able to afford these private services can take advantage of them.

Current Health Issues

Two medical problems which are the focus of much research and discussion today are AIDS and alcoholism. Although both are treated as medical problems, their cause and solution are outside medical practice and within social relationships. AIDS is a disease in the classical sense since it can be traced back to a virus. However alcoholism is not. Yet medical science treats both problems within the same set of procedures, that is, by looking for a drug to cure them.

AIDS

In 1981 physicians in New York and San Francisco began to see homosexual men dying from either a rare form of cancer known as Kaposi's Sarcoma or from previously non-fatal infections. The names first given to their condition, Gay Compromise Syndrome or Gay-Related Immunodeficiency Disease, had grave social, psychological and medical consequences for homosexuals. Soon it was found that not only male homosexuals, but also women engaging in anal intercourse, drug addicts using intravenous injections, hemophiliacs receiving blood transfusions, and Haitians also contracted the disease (Thomas 1983, 42-47).[4] The name was then changed to Acquired Immune Deficiency Syndrome, or AIDS.

Although some groups see AIDS as a divine punishment meted out to "deviants," this view is of course preposterous. Diseases make no moral judgements, and no humane, thinking person would say that any individual or group "deserves" to get a disease.

Even though there is now mass hysteria about contracting AIDS, it is very difficult to catch, for the HIV (Human Immunodeficiency Virus) does not appear to be highly contagious. The virus is not spread by casual contact: according to the latest information, you cannot get the virus from telephones, toilet seats, swimming pools, whirlpools, buses or trains, hugging or sharing glasses or dishes. AIDS is transmissible through unprotected (i.e. without a condom) sexual contact and through blood.

While many people now have the virus, only a small number of these people are diagnosed as having AIDS. Therefore, having the virus, or the supposed predisposition to AIDS, does not mean you will necessarily get the disease.

> While it seems clear that there is some link between AIDS and HTLV-3, other explanations of this relationship cannot be ruled out. It is possible, for example, that some unknown Factor X leads to infection with the HTLV-3 virus, which in turn causes AIDS; alternatively, some Factor X might cause both AIDS and HTLV-3 infection. (Freudenberg 1985, 29)

At the biological level of explanation, a disease is thought to have a cause, and once this cause is eliminated or a way is found to intervene in the cause/effect process, then the disease will be eliminated. In fact, this is not true for all diseases; hypertension is a good example. Some individuals may have a supposed cause (say, a virus) within them, yet do not contract the disease, and vice versa. "Some individuals with AIDS show no evidence of HTLV-3 . . . [the virus] could be isolated from only 50% of the patients with AIDS and 85% of the patients with the syndrome called AIDS Related Complex" (Cohen 1985, 10).

Furthermore, even though this model places much emphasis on the cause of the disease, solutions tend to focus not on prevention but on eliminating the symptoms of the disease. The search for a single factor or vaccine as the cause or cure for AIDS may in fact be useless, since there are already new strains of the virus showing up in the heterosexual population (Veitch 1988a; Deer 1987).

Since AIDS is known to have a limited way of spreading from one individual to another, would it not be more beneficial to spend money on education to stop the spread of the disease? Yet some governments find this difficult, since they are afraid of being seen as condoning homosexual or extramarital sexual activity. Yet less money is spent on education than on research: the Mulroney Conservative government had spent $2 million on AIDS research by 1985 (Canada 1985a). As of 1988, the Canadian Health Minister, Jake Epp, has adopted a wait-and-see attitude toward AIDS and advocates still more money for research.

Alcoholism

It was estimated that in 1979 there were approximately 630,000 alcoholics in Canada, and 2.5 male alcoholics for every female alcoholic.[5] We must understand that the social problem of alcoholism is not restricted to the native peoples of Canada, but is turning up in all groups in Canadian society. In 1976 a majority of problem alcoholics, 59%, were English, while other ethnic groups (French, Indian and others) each made up less than 20% of the total (Canada 1981b). There are many deaths in Canada every year which are in some way related to the consumption of alcohol (Canada 1981b, 16):

i)   Direct causes of death related to alcohol:
        Cirrhosis of the Liver
        Alcoholism
        Alcoholic Psychosis and Poisoning
ii) Indirect causes of death related to alcohol:
        Motor Vehicle Accidents
        Suicide
        Fall
        Fire and Drowning
        Homicide
iii) Other related causes of death:
        Heart Condition
        Cancer
        Respiratory Condition

In Canada the federal government publishes data on the amount of alcohol consumed weekly by the population and the type of drinker by province and work. However, this information does not indicate how and when alcohol is consumed, or if there is a relation between the amount drunk and the number of alcoholics (Abelson, Paddon and Strohmenger 1983, 26). Alcohol consumption has become not only a social problem but also an economic problem felt by individuals and families. Many hospital beds are filled by the problems created by alcohol abuse. On the other hand, governments collect a great amount of money from the sales tax on alcohol. Today, alcoholism is popularly called a "disease" (Fitzpatrick 1982, 9-10), but is it *really* a disease? Is there a germ or genetic factor which causes this condition? How do we benefit, socially or medically, by calling it a disease? What type of treatment does it demand and where is the focus of the problem? Does the clinical method of medical intervention disguise the causes of this problem? These are all important questions, since the concept of "disease" is creeping into our language and being applied loosely to various *behaviours*. Treating alcoholism as a disease may make a social problem a medical one, but it does not cure the problem.

Heavy drinking is not necessarily alcoholism, so how do we distinguish between the two? According to Fitzpatrick (1982, 9):

> ... most people would argue that essential to a definition [of alcoholism] is ... whether drinking causes difficulties for the individual at home or work. Also important are judgments as to whether heavy drinking is "out of control". However, if one accepts such arguments, social criteria are being brought into the definition of disease, which considerably extend the term beyond its orthodox medical usage.... Although few doctors seem to blame the alcoholic in a moral sense, they nevertheless feel irritated about their involvement in a problem where patients often deny their illness and are poorly motivated to cooperate in treatment. Doctors feel there are few effective medical remedies available for what they see as a complex social problem.

Alcoholism is not universal: it is a cultural product. For instance, Italy and France both have high rates of alcohol consumption and production, and are fairly similar cultures. Yet in France alcoholism is a national problem and in Italy it is not (Jones and Jones 1975, 97). In some societies alcohol has been integrated into social life, and in others it has become a crutch to help overcome social, psychological and economic problems (Jones and Jones 1975, 96). Rates of alcoholism may depend on the cultural role of alcohol and the individual tolerance of those who drink: certain groups, families or individuals may have a lower than average tolerance for alcohol.

If alcoholism is classified as a disease, a condition to be medically treated, then it is not the "fault" of the individual since it is out of his control. The medical model lifts the responsibility from both the individual and the society; the individual is no longer the focus of condemnation (his disease is) and the society is neutral (Zola 1972, 490). A certain amount of sympathy is given to those affected by the disease. According to the disease model, individuals must be treated medically after they become alcoholics. The question of the individual's responsibility for his behaviour is tossed aside, since biology is seen as the root of the problem.

This perspective has found its way into the current biological determinism of certain sociologists (Kitcher 1985).

Even though alcoholics are dependent on alcohol to the degree that they show a noticeable change in mental and bodily health and in their social relationships, we still cannot call alcoholism a disease since the condition is not caused by something within the individual.

Unfortunately, much is still unknown about alcoholism. There is the question of why people start to drink and why drinking is a behavioural option. Also, why is alcohol used as an excuse for deviant or illegal acts? These questions are not receiving the attention they should, because the biomedical model is taking over. Zola (1972 and 1975) asserts that medical explanations have replaced the religious and legal explanations of behaviour, and that this is not a move from morality to science but to a new type of scientific morality which has certain consequences for our lives.

What are the consequences of having medical science deal with this social problem, and what are the situations which cause people to drink in excessive amounts? What is it that people are escaping from and why is alcohol a vehicle for escape? These questions cannot be answered by medical science.

There is no immediate solution to the problem of alcoholism. Alcoholism may be an illness but it is certainly not a disease which manipulates a person's behaviour. If the real cause of alcoholism is stress or tension, then what is the cause of this – work, family, school, the threat of nuclear war?

Concentration on individual ills forces us to help the individuals who are victims. However, we have to acknowledge that treating individuals is superficial because it ignores the larger social issues involved in the production and use of alcohol in our society. We should blame neither the alcohol nor human biology for alcoholism. The elimination of alcohol is not the answer either, since there are cultures which have high rates of alcohol use without the high rates of alcoholism. What we should do is consider prevention, not through medicine, but by transforming the social conditions and relationships which reinforce the continuance of alcoholism.

Summary

There are two main points in this chapter. First, patients and their supporters have to organize themselves to put the patient back into patient care; those not willing to fight for changes within the health-care system are seeking alternatives which focus on the patient instead of the disease. Second, major threats to individuals and society, whether they be viral or behavioural, cannot be treated by medicine alone. Social problems need social answers.

Notes

1. This is often the case when the physician does not know which antibiotic would best suit the situation. These antibiotics are usually samples provided to doctors by drug companies.
2. Some medical researchers are now finding that "alternative therapists who prescribe meditation and Yoga for AIDS patients may be on the right track" since stress plays a major part in the move from the HIV virus to AIDS (Veitch 1988b).
3. This connection will be familiar to sociology students who have read C. Wright Mills' *The Sociological Imagination*.
4. Sexually active gays may encounter the virus HIV (formerly called HTLV-3) more frequently and therefore may overtax their immune systems by repeated infections. Anal intercourse results in intestinal abrasions, and breaks in the mucosal surface serve as pools for viruses and other bacterial material. There is evidence to suggest that amyl and butyl nitrate inhalants ("poppers") and other recreational drugs (cocaine and amphetamines), used by some homosexuals to enhance orgasm, act as immunosuppressive agents. Other weakeners of the immune system include petrochemical-based lubricants. In addition, the social stress from stigmatization of homosexuals may weaken the immune system.
5. The rate of alcoholism in Canada is about average for Western countries.

Glossary

Acute

Having a short and relatively severe course (pertaining to a disease or illness).

Antibiotic

A drug that inhibits the growth of bacteria and some moulds.

Antibody

A kind of protein made by the body to fight off invading micro-organisms or other foreign matter.

Antigen

Any substance that the body regards as foreign or dangerous.

Bacteria

One-celled micro-organisms that may cause disease.

Birthing Rooms

Hospital rooms designed to resemble a comfortable home environment and used for giving birth.

Brand-Name Drug

A drug or preparation having a company trade mark. Pharmaceutical companies argue that brand-name drugs are better because they contain special ingredients to assist the primary drug. Brand-name drugs are much more expensive than generic drugs. (Note that a given generic drug can have several different brand names.)

Carcinogenic

Cancer-producing.

Cardiovascular Disease

A disease of the circulatory system (heart and blood vessels)

Cause

In epidemiology, if the presence or absence of some factor affects the chances of some event occurring, then the factor is the "cause" of that event.

Cerebrovascular Disease

A disease of the blood vessels of the brain and its covering membranes.

Chemotherapy

The treatment of disease by administering chemicals that, in theory, affect the causative organism unfavorably. (Note that these chemicals may also adversely affect the patient.)

Cholesterol

A fatty compound made by the body and found in food; an excess of cholesterol impairs the cardiovascular system.

Chronic

Long and continued (pertaining to illness)

Cohort

All people in the same age group.

Communicable Disease

A disease that can be passed from one person to another, directly or indirectly.

Concept

A notion or idea on a lower level of abstraction than a theory.

Coronary Heart Disease

A disease resulting from changes in the arteries supplying the heart and the subsequent interference with blood flow.

Debilitating

Producing weakness.

Demography

The study of human populations in relation to their size, structure and development.

Division of Labour

The division of the work process into a group of parts, each of which is done by a separate individual or group.

Drug

Any substance, natural or man-made, that alters an individual's physical, mental, emotional or social condition.

Drug Dependence

A state resulting from the interaction of a living organism with a drug.

Empirical Knowledge

Information about the world gained through the physical senses.

Endemic

Always in existence in a given area (pertaining to a disease).

Epidemic

The sudden outbreak of infectious disease that spreads rapidly through the population.

Epidemiology

The study of how and why diseases are distributed within a population.

Episiotomy

A surgical incision to enlarge the outlet of the birth canal; done to prevent tearing.

Etiology

The study of causation. (Also spelled *aetiology*.)

Euthanasia

The practice of allowing or painlessly speeding the death of a person with an incurable disease.

Fecundity

The physical possibility of having a child; usually applies to women between the ages of 16 and 44.

Foetus

An embryo between the fifth week of pregnancy and delivery.

Generic Drug
A drug or preparation named according to its chemical makeup.

Hospice
A place that provides palliative care and support by addressing the spiritual, emotional, physical, economic and medical needs of the terminally ill.

Iatrogenesis
Sickness produced by a physician.

Ideology
A pattern of concepts and beliefs that provides a total explanation of complex social phenomena.

Infection
The entry and development or multiplication of an infectious agent in a living organism.

Immune
Having resistance to a disease, so that one may be exposed to the disease without catching it.

Immunization
Providing a person with the ability to resist infection or disease.

Incidence Rate
The measure of the new cases of a disease or illness during a given period.

Ischemic Disease
A disease affecting the flow of blood through the body; a constriction or blockage of a vessel.

Lamaze Method
A method that conditions the pregnant woman to dissociate labour contractions from pain and teaches her to respond to these contractions with a set of learned breathing patterns.

Labelling
The process by which people classify and categorize social behaviour and other individuals.

Lay Midwives

Non-medically trained midwives who do the same tasks as nurse-midwives. Lay midwives are not licensed to practise in Canada.

Lifestyle

A way of behaving, including the way we attempt to control our health.

Life Chances

A person's access to the supply of goods, living conditions and life experiences.

Menarche

First menstruation.

Menopause

The cessation of menstruation.

Model

A simple system or framework that can be applied to a more complex theme.

Morbidity

Refers to the amount of illness or disease in a given area.

Mortality

Refers to death.
Infant mortality: deaths under 1 year of age.
Neonatal mortality: deaths under 28 days of age.
Post-neonatal mortality: deaths between 4 weeks and 1 year.
Perinatal mortality: foetal deaths of 28 or more weeks' gestation, plus infant deaths under 7 days.

Nosocomial

Hospital-induced (applies to infections).

Nurse-Midwives

Registered nurses trained in obstetrics and able to recognize any abnormality in pregnancy, labour and babies. They can deliver babies, but are not licensed to practise in Canada.

Over-the-Counter Drugs

Medications available without a prescription.

Palliative Care

Medical care aimed at relieving or alleviating pain and suffering, rather than curing. This type of care is given to the chronically or terminally ill, and to the aged.

Population

De jure definition: population actually present at the time of enumeration.
De facto definition: population usually present in a given area.

Population at Risk

All those to whom an event could have happened, whether it did or not.

Prescription Drugs

Medications available only from a pharmacist upon orders (or prescription) from a doctor.

Prevalence Rate

A measurement of the total cases of a disease or illness prevailing at a given time.

Profession

Autonomous occupation demanding highly specialized knowledge and skills.

Prognosis

Prediction of the course and end of a disease

Rate

Computed or estimated quantity of something, usually as forming a basis for calculating other quantities or sums.

Ratio

The relationship of one number to another. e.g. the sex ratio is the number of males for every 100 females in the population.

Risk Factor

Any particular factor that increases the risk of some event happening.

Somatic

Of or relating to the body.

Stratification

The ranking of families, persons or kinship groups in a society relative to each other, according to prestige, power and property.

Symptomatology

The study of signs or symptoms of an illness or disease.

Taxonomy

The classification of material under study; the study of classification systems.

Toxic

Pertaining to poison; poisonous.

Virus

Extremely small micro-organism that may cause disease.

Bibliography

Abelson, J., P. Paddon, and C. Strohmenger
  1983   *Perspectives on Health*. Ottawa: Statistics Canada.

Alexander, C.
  1986   "The Cultural Basis of Well-Being." *Healthsharing* 7, no. 3.

Allentuck, A.
  1978   *Who Speaks for the Patient*. Don Mills, Ontario: Burns and MacEachern.

American Funeral Director
  1984   "Decline in Autopsies Called Deplorable." Vol. 107, no. 7.

Anderson, A.B. and J.S. Frideres
  1981   *Ethnicity in Canada*. Toronto: Butterworths.

Anderson, J.A.
  1986   "Ethnicity and Illness Experience." *Social Science and Medicine* 22, no. 11.

Andreopoulos, S. (ed.)
  1975   *National Health Insurance*. New York: Wiley.

Anthony, W. and M. Jansen
  1984   "Predicting the Vocational Capacity of the Chronically Mentally Ill." *American Psychologist* 39, no. 5.

Antony, W.
  1985   "Sensitive to the Difficulties of Employers? Safety and Health in Manitoba." *Canadian Dimension* 19, no. 3.

Appelbaum, P. and L. Roth
  1983   "Patients Who Refuse Treatment in Medical Hospitals." *Journal of the American Medical Association* 250, no. 10.

Apple, D.
  1960   "How Laymen Define Illness." *Journal of Health and Human Behaviour* 1.

Ardell, D.B.
  1985   "The History and the Future of Wellness." *Health Values* 9, no. 6.

Armitage, A.
   1979   *Social Welfare in Canada: Ideas and Realities.* Toronto: McClelland and Stewart.

Armstrong, D.
   1980   *An Outline of Sociology as Applied to Medicine.* Bristol: John Wright and Sons.

Armstrong, D.
   1983   *An Outline of Sociology as Applied to Medicine*, 2nd ed. London: Wright-PSG.

Armstrong, D.
   1984   "The Patient's View." *Social Science and Medicine* 18, no. 9.

Armstrong, J.
   1987   "Prescribed Drugs Linked to 20% of Emergencies." *Winnipeg Free Press*, 2 March.

Armstrong, P. and H. Armstrong
   1983   *A Working Majority.* Ottawa: Canadian Advisory Council on the Status of Women.

Arney, W.
   1982   *Power and the Profession of Obstetrics.* Chicago: University of Chicago Press.

Attman, L.K., T.J. Thom, and M. Feinleib
   1984   "Declining Autopsy Rates and Diagnosis of Myocardial Infarction." *Journal of the American Medical Association* 251, no. 17.

Badgley, R.F.
   1976   "The Sociology of Health in Canada." *Social Science and Medicine* 10, no. 1.

Badgley, R.F. and R.W. Hetherington
   1961   "Medical Sociology: A Selected Canadian Bibliography." *Canadian Medical Association Journal* 85.

Badgley, R.F. and S. Wolfe
   1967   *Doctor's Strike.* Toronto: Macmillan.

Baltzan, M.
   1973   "Report's Data and Interpretation Suspect." *Canadian Medical Association Journal* 109, October.

Banagale, R.
   1984   "Iatrogenous Complications in the Fetus and Newborn." *American Journal of Diseases of Children* 138, July.

Banta, H. and S. Thacker
   1979   *Costs and Benefits of Electronic Fetal Monitoring.* Washington: Department of Health, Education and Welfare.

Barer, M.
1981   *Community Health Centres and Hospital Costs in Ontario.* Toronto: Ontario Economic Council.

Barer, M., R. Evans, and G. Stoddart
1979   *Controlling Health Care Costs by Direct Charges to Patients: Snare or Delusion.* Toronto: Ontario Economic Council.

Barr, J.
1983   "Physicians' Views of Patients in Prepaid Group Practice: Reasons for Visits to HMOs." *Journal of Health and Social Behaviour* 24, no. 3.

Barrington, E.
1985   *Midwifery Is Catching.* Toronto: NC Press.

Bassuk, E.L.
1986   "The Rest Cure: Repetition or Resolution of Victorian Women's Conflicts." In S.R. Suleiman (ed.), *The Female Body in Western Culture.* Cambridge, Mass.: Harvard University Press.

Bates, B.
1978   "Doctor and Nurse: Changing Roles and Relations." *New England Journal of Medicine* 283, July.

Beaujot, R. and K. McQuillan
1982   *Growth and Dualism.* Toronto: Gage Publishing.

Beavis, S.
1988   "Study Finds Stress Hits Most Workers." *The Guardian*, 29 February.

Belle, E., T. D'Souza, J. Zarzour, M. Lemieux, and C. Wong
1979   "Hospital Epidemics of Scabies: Diagnosis and Control." *Canadian Journal of Public Health* 70, no. 2.

Benn, M. and R. Richardson
1984   "Uneasy Freedom: Women's Experiences of Contraception." *Women's Studies International Forum* 7, no. 4.

Bennet, G.
1987   *The Wound and the Doctor.* London: Secker and Warburg.

Bennett, J. and J. Krasney
1980   "Health Care in Canada." Parts 1-6. *The Financial Post.* 26 March.

Berger, J.W.
1980   *Report on the Advisory Commission on Indian and Inuit Health Consultation.* Ottawa: Minister of Supply and Services.

Berger, P. and T. Luckmann
1967   *The Social Construction of Reality.* New York: Doubleday.

Berliner, H.S.
 1975   "A Larger Perspective on the Flexner Report." *International Journal of Health Services* 5, no. 4.

Berliner, H.S.
 1977   "Emerging Ideologies in Medicine." *Review of Radical Political Economics* 9, no. 1.

Besharah, A.
 1985   "Jury Recommends Legalization, Recognition of Midwifery in Ontario." *The Canadian Nurse*, September.

Best, M.
 1982   "Indians: Victims of Failed Policy." *The Winnipeg Sun*, 24 October.

Billette, A.
 1977   "Les inégalités sociales de mortalité au Québec." *Recherches sociographiques* XVIII, no. 3.

Billette, A. and G. Hill
 1977   *Inégalités sociales de mortalité au Canada.* Ottawa: Department of National Health and Welfare.

Black, E.
 1981   "Dealing With the Doctors: The Canadian Experience." *Monthly Review*, September.

Black, N. et al. (eds.)
 1984   *Health and Disease, A Reader.* London: Open University Press.

Blakiston's Gould Medical Dictionary
 1979   Toronto: McGraw-Hill.

Blane, D.
 1982   "Inequalities and Social Class." In D.L. Patrick and G. Scambler (eds.), *Sociology as Applied to Medicine.* London: Bailliere Tindall.

Blishen, B.R. and W.K. Carroll
 1978   "Sex Differences in a Socio-Economic Index for Occupations in Canada." *The Canadian Review of Sociology and Anthropology* 15, no. 3.

Bloch, M. and J. Parry
 1982   *Death and the Regeneration of Life.* Cambridge: Cambridge University Press.

Blomquist, A.
 1979   *The Health Care Business.* Vancouver: The Fraser Institute.

Boase, J.
 1982   "Regulation and the Paramedical Professions: An Interest Group Study." *Canadian Public Administration* 25, no. 3.

Bohuslawsky, M.
  1987   "Shades of Gray." Part 5. *Winnipeg Free Press*, 22 April.

Bolaria, B. Singh and H. Dickinson (eds.)
  1988   *Sociology of Health Care in Canada*. Toronto: Harcourt Brace Jovanovich.

Bond, J. and S. Bond
  1986   *Sociology and Health Care*. London: Churchill Livingstone.

Borges, S.
  1986   "A Feminist Critique of Scientific Ideology: An Analysis of Two Doctor-Patient Encounters." In S. Fisher and A. Todd (eds.), *Discourse and Institutional Authority*. Norwood, N.J.: Ablex.

Boston Women's Health Collective
  1984   *The New Our Bodies, Ourselves*. New York: Simon and Schuster.

Brady, P.D.
  1984   "Contradictions and Consequences: The Social and Health Status of Canada's Registered Indian Population." In J.A. Fry (ed.), *Contradictions in Canadian Society*. Toronto: Wiley and Sons.

Brandejs, J.
  1973   "Report Fails to Deal with Incentive Issue for Clinics Physicians." *Canadian Medical Association Journal* 109, October.

Brandon, V.
  1984   "Medibucks." *Canadian Dimension* 18, no. 2.

Braunstein, J. and G. Silverman
  1981   "The Physician-Patient Relationship." In J. Braunstein and R. Toister (eds.), *Medical Applications of the Behavioral Sciences*. Chicago: Year Book Medical Publishers.

Braunstein, J. and R. Toister (eds.)
  1981   *Medical Applications of the Behavioral Sciences*. Chicago: Year Book Medical Publishers.

Braverman, H.
  1974   *Labour and Monopoly Capital*. New York: Monthly Review Press.

Brenner, M.H.
  1979   "Mortality and the National Economy." *The Lancet*, 15 September.

Breton, R.
  1964   "Institutional Completeness of Ethnic Communities and the Personal Relations of Immigrants." *American Journal of Sociology* LXX, no. 2.

Brett, B., W.C. Taylor, and D.W. Spady
   1986   "The Northwest Territories Perinatal and Infant Mortality Study." In Shepard and Itoh (eds.), *Circumpolar Health*. Toronto: University of Toronto Press.

Brodeur, P.
   1985   "Annals of Asbestos." *The New Yorker*. Parts I-IV, 10 June, 17 June, 24 June and 1 July.

Bruyer, J.
   1981   *The Manitoba Native Indian Mother and Child*. Ottawa: Community Task Force on Maternal and Child Health.

Buck, C.
   1985   "Beyond Lalonde—Creating Health." *Canadian Journal of Public Health* 76, Supp. no. 1.

Bulkley, B. and R. Ross
   1978   "Coronary-Artery Bypass Surgery: It Works, But Why?" *Annals of Internal Medicine* 88, no. 6.

Bullough, B. and V. Bullough
   1975   "Sex Discrimination in Health Care." *Nursing Outlook* 23, no. 1.

Burtch, B.
   1986   "Community Midwifery and State Measures: The New Midwifery in British Columbia." *Contemporary Crisis* 10, no. 4.

Canada
   1969   *Task Force Reports on the Cost of Health Care Services in Canada*. Ottawa: Department of Health and Welfare.

Canada
   1971   *Census of Canada 1971: Labour Force by Occupation*. Catalogue no. 94-788. Ottawa: Statistics Canada.

Canada
   1975   *Occupational Distribution of Employment: Canada and Provinces*. Ottawa: Statistics Canada.

Canada
   1978   *Nursing in Canada: Canadian Nursing Statistics*. Ottawa: Statistics Canada.

Canada
   1979   *Indian Health Discussion Paper*. Ottawa: Health and Welfare Canada, Medical Services Branch.

Canada
   1980a   *Indian Conditions: A Survey*. Ottawa: Department of Indian Affairs and Northern Development.

Canada
1980b *Mortality Atlas of Canada: Vol. 1: Cancer.* Ottawa: Minister of National Health and Welfare.

Canada
1980c *Mortality Atlas of Canada: Vol. 2: General Mortality.* Ottawa: Minister of National Health and Welfare.

Canada
1981a *The Health of Canadians.* Ottawa: Health and Welfare Canada.

Canada
1981b *A Special Report on Alcohol Statistics.* Ottawa: Health and Welfare Canada.

Canada
1983a The Canada Health Act.

Canada
1983b *Causes of Death. Vital Statistics, Vol. IV.* Ottawa: Statistics Canada.

Canada
1983c *In Sickness and Health: Health Statistics at a Glance.* Ottawa: Statistics Canada.

Canada
1983d *Medicare: The Public Good and Private Practice.* Ottawa: National Council of Welfare.

Canada
1983e *Mortality. Vital Statistics, Vol. III.* Ottawa: Statistics Canada.

Canada
1983f *National Health Expenditure in Canada, 1970-1982.* Health and Welfare Canada.

Canada
1983g *Registered Nurses Data Services.* Ottawa: Statistics Canada.

Canada
1984a *Canada Health Manpower Inventory.* Ottawa: Health and Welfare Canada.

Canada
1984b *Charting Canadian Incomes: 1951-1981.* Ottawa: Statistics Canada.

Canada
1984c *Hospital Morbidity: 1979-80 and 1980-81.* Ottawa: Statistics Canada.

Canada
1984d *Sixty-Five and Older.* Report by the National Council of Welfare on Incomes of Aged. Ottawa: National Council of Welfare.

Canada
1985a *Aids in Canada: What You Should Know.* Ottawa: Health and Welfare Canada.

Canada
1985b *Poverty Profile 1985.* Ottawa: National Council of Welfare.

Canada
1985c Taxation Returns by Province and Occupation. Catalogue 44. Ottawa: Revenue Canada.

Canada
1987 *Social Trends.* Winter. Ottawa: Statistics Canada.

Canada Year Book
1985 Ottawa: Statistics Canada.

Canadian Council on Social Development
1984 *Not Enough: The Meaning and Measurement of Poverty in Canada.* Ottawa: The Canadian Council on Social Development.

Canadian Medical Association
1982 Canadian Medical Association Policy Summary. *CMAJ.* 134, 25 June.

Cann, B. et al.
1987 "Midwifery: A Discussion Paper." Winnipeg: Manitoba Advisory Council on the Status of Women.

Carlson, R.
1985 "Healthy People." *Canadian Journal of Public Health* 76, supplement 1.

Carr, T.
1981 "Environmental Health in the Keewatin." *University of Manitoba Medical Journal* 51, no. 1.

Chappell, N. and N. Clovill
1981 "Medical Schools as Agents of Socialization." *Canadian Review of Sociology and Anthropology* 18, no. 1.

Chappell, N., L. Strain, and A. Blandford
1986 *Aging and Health Care: A Social Perspective.* Toronto: W.B. Saunders

Chenier, H.
1982 *Reproductive Hazards of Work.* Ottawa: Advisory Council on the Status of Women.

Cleland, V.
1971 "Sex Discrimination: Nursing's Most Pervasive Problem." *American Journal of Nursing* 71, no. 2.

Clement, W.
1983 *Class, Power and Property.* Toronto: Methuen.

Coates, D.
1969 "Is There a Power Elite in Canadian Psychiatry?" *Canadian Psychiatric Association Journal* 14, no. 2.

Coburn, D.
1978 "Work and General Psychological Well-Being." *International Journal of Health Services* 8, no. 3.

Coburn, D.
1980 "Patients' Rights: A New Deal in Health Care." *Canadian Forum*, May.

Coburn, D., C. D'Arcy, G. Torrance, and P. New (eds.)
1981 *Health and Canadian Society*, 1st and 2nd ed. Toronto:
1987 Fitzhenry and Whiteside.

Coburn, D. and C.L. Biggs
1987 "Legitimation or Medicalization? The Case of Chiropractic in Canada." In D. Coburn et al. (eds.), *Health and Canadian Society*, 2nd ed. Toronto: Fitzhenry and Whiteside.

Coburn, D. and C. Pope
1974 "Socioeconomic Status and Preventive Health Behaviour." *Journal of Health and Social Behaviour* 15, June.

Coburn, J.
1987 " 'I See and Am Silent.' A Short History of Nursing in Ontario." In D. Coburn et al. (eds.) *Health and Canadian Society*, 2nd ed. Toronto: Fitzhenry and Whiteside.

Cochrane, D.
1972 *Effectiveness and Efficiency, Random Reflections on Health Services*. London: Nuffield Provincial Hospitals Trust.

Cockerham, W.C.
1986 *Medical Sociology*. Englewood Cliffs, N.J.: Prentice Hall.

Coe, R.M.
1978 *Sociology of Medicine*, 2nd ed. Toronto: McGraw-Hill.

Cohen, N. and L. Estner
1983 *Silent Knife*. S. Hadley: Bergin and Garvey.

Cohen, R.
1985 "AIDS: The Impending Quarantine." *Health/Pac Bulletin* 16, no. 4.

Conn, M. and R. Fox
1980 "Undoing Medical Conditioning." *Healthsharing*, Fall.

Conrad, P. and R. Kern (eds.)
1981 *The Sociology of Health and Illness*, 1st and 2nd ed. New York:
1986 St. Martin's Press.

Conrad, P. and J. Schneider
1986 "Professionalization, Monopoly and the Structure of Medical Practice." In P. Conrad and R. Kern (eds.), *The Sociology of Health and Illness*, 2nd ed. New York: St. Martin's Press.

Coombes, R. and L.J. Goldman
1973 "Maintenance and Discontinuity of Coping Mechanisms in an Intensive Care Unit." *Social Problems* 20, no. 3.

Cooper, B. and C. Gaus
1979 *Medical Technology.* Washington: Department of Health, Education and Welfare.

Coreil, J. and J.S. Levin
1984 "A Critique of the Life Style Concept in Public Health Educa-
-85 tion." *International Quarterly of Community Health and Education* 5, no. 2.

Coulson, M. and C. Riddell
1980 *Approaching Sociology.* London: Routledge and Kegan Paul.

Crichton, A., J. Lawerence, and S. Lee (eds.)
1984 *The Canadian Health Care System.* Vols. 1-5. Ottawa: Canadian Hospital Association.

Crowe, K.
1974 *A History of the Original Peoples of Northern Canada.* Toronto: Queen's University Press.

Currer, C. and M. Stacey (eds.)
1986 *Concepts of Health, Illness and Disease.* Leamington Spa: Berg.

Czerny, M. and J. Swift
1984 *Getting Started on Social Analysis in Canada.* Toronto: Between the Lines.

D'Arcy, C. and M. Siddique
1985 "Unemployment and Health: An Analysis of 'Canada Health Survey' Data." *International Journal of Health Services* 15, no. 4.

D'Arcy, C. and M. Siddique
1987 "Health and Unemployment: Findings from a National Survey." In D. Coburn et al. (eds.), *Health and Canadian Society*, 2nd ed. Toronto: Fitzhenry and Whiteside.

Davis, D.L.
1984 "Medical Misinformation: Communication Between Outport Newfoundland Women and Their Physicians." *Social Science and Medicine* 18, no. 3.

Davis, K.
1984 "Women as Patients: A Problem for Sex Differences Research." *Women's Studies International Forum* 7, no. 4.

Davis, K. and W. Moore
  1945   "Some Principles of Stratification." *American Sociological Review* 10, no. 2.

Davis, K. and C. Schoen
  1978   *Health and the War on Poverty.* Washington: Brookings Institute.

Deber, R. and P. Leatt
  1986   "Technology Acquisition in Ontario Hospitals." Paper presented at the Third Canadian Conference on Health Economics, Winnipeg.

Deer, B.
  1987   "Scientists Fear Dangers from New AIDS Strain." *The London Times*, 13 September.

Denton, J.
  1978   *Medical Sociology.* Boston: Houghton Miffin.

de Pouvourville, G. and M. Renaud
  1985   "Hospital System Management in France and Canada: National Pluralism and Provincial Centralism." *Social Science and Medicine* 20, no. 2.

Devitt, J.E.
  1985   "Screening for Breast Cancer: Current Status, Problems and Prospects." *Canadian Family Physician* 31, Jan.

Dickenson, H. and P. Brady
  1984   "The Labour Process and the Transformation of Health Care Delivery." In J. Fry (ed.), *Contradictions in Canadian Society.* Toronto: Wiley and Sons.

Dilley, J., H. Ochitill, M. Perl, and P. Volberding
  1985   "Findings in Psychiatric Consultations with Patients with AIDS." *American Journal of Psychiatry* 124, no. 4.

Doyal, L.
  1979   *The Political Economy of Health.* London: Pluto Press.

Doyal, L.
  1983   "Women, Health and the Sexual Division of Labour." *Critical Social Policy*, no. 7

Doyal, L. and M.A. Elston
  1986   "Women, Health and Medicine." In V. Beechey and E. Whitelegg (eds.), *Women in Britain Today.* London: Open University Press.

Dreitzel, H.P.
  1971   *The Social Organization of Health.* London: Collier-Macmillan.

Dubos, R.
  1959   *Mirage of Health*. New York: Perennial Library.

Dubos, R.
  1979   "Medicine Evolving." In D. Sobel (ed.), *Ways of Health*. New York: Harcourt Brace Jovanovich.

Duff, R. and A. Hollingshead
  1968   *Sickness and Society*, New York: Harper and Row.

Dumas, J.
  1984   *Report on Demographic Situation in Canada: Current Demographic Analysis*. Catalogue no. 91-209. Ottawa: Statistics Canada.

Durkheim, E.
  1952   *Suicide*. Glencoe: Free Press.

Egan, H.
  1974   "How It Feels to Be a Ventilator Patient." *Respiratory Care* 19, no. 4.

Ehrenreich, B. and J. Ehrenreich
  1973   "Hospital Workers: A Case Study in the 'New Working Class'." *Monthly Review*, January.

Ehrenreich, B. and J. Ehrenreich
  1975   "Hospital Workers: Class Conflicts in the Making." *International Journal of Health Services* 5, no. 1.

Ehrenreich, B. and J. Ehrenreich
  1978   "Medicine and Social Control," in J. Ehrenreich (ed.), *The Cultural Crisis of Modern Medicine*. New York: Monthly Review Press.

Ehrenreich, B. and D. English
  1978   *For Her Own Good*. New York: Anchor Press.

Ehrenreich, J. (ed.)
  1978   *The Cultural Crisis of Modern Medicine*. New York: Monthly Review Press.

Eisenburg, L. and A. Kleinman (eds.)
  1981   *The Relevance of Social Science for Medicine*. London: Reidel.

el-Guebaly, N.
  1984   "The Interaction with Non-Medical Professions: The Canadian Psychiatric Association's Guidelines." *Canadian Journal of Psychiatry* 29, March.

Engel, G.L.
  1977   "The Need for a New Medical Model." *Science* 196, no. 4286.

England
  1988   *Stress at Work*. London: Labour Research Department.

Engman, K.
1986 "Two Doctors Ordered to Repay $128,405 in Medical Billings." *Winnipeg Free Press*, 11 July.

Engman, K.
1987a "HSC Considers Bed Closing in Planning Cost-Cutting Tack." *Winnipeg Free Press*, 16 February.

Engman, K.
1987b "MDs Pay Called Abysmal." *Winnipeg Free Press*, 8 June.

Esser, P. and R. Johnston
1984 *Technology of Nuclear Magnetic Resonance*. New York: The Society of Nuclear Medicine Inc.

Evans, D.A., M.R. Block, E.R. Steinburg, and A.M. Penrose
1986 "Frame and Heuristics in Doctor-Patient Discourse." *Social Science and Medicine* 22, no. 10.

Evans, R.G.
1973 "Supplier-Induced Demand: Some Empirical Evidence and Implication." In M. Perlman (ed.), *The Economics of Health and Medical Care*. Edinburgh: Clark.

Evans, R.G.
1984 *Strained Mercy: The Economics of Canadian Health Care*. Toronto: Butterworths.

Evans, R.G.
1987 "Finding the Levers, Finding the Courage: Lessons from Cost Containment in North America." *Journal of Health Politics, Policy and Law* 11, no. 4.

Evans, R.G., D. Roch, and D. Pascoe
1986 "Defensive Reticulation: Physician Supply Increases and Practice Pattern Changes in Manitoba, 1971-1981." Paper presented at the Third Canadian Conference on Health Economics, Winnipeg.

Eyer, J.
1977 "Does Unemployment Cause the Death Rate Peak in Each Business Cycle." *International Journal of Health Services* 7, no. 4.

Fairfax, M.
1982 "Canada: Higher Fees, Lower Wages." *Health/Pac Bulletin* 13, no. 4.

Family Planning Perspectives
1981 "Legal Abortion, Family Planning Services Largest Factors in Reducing U.S. Neonatal Mortality." Vol. 13, no. 2.

Fawzy, F. et al.
1981 "Preventing Nursing Burnout." *General Hospital Psychiatry* 13, no. 2.

Ferguson, C.
   1975   "Chemical Abuse in the North." *University of Manitoba Medical Journal* 45, no. 3.

Ferguson, G.
   1985   "Where's the Credibility in Hospital Administrators." *Canadian Medical Association Journal* 132, no. 3.

Ferriman, A.
   1988   "Op a Good Thing?" *The Observer*, 31 July, p. 36.

Fidell, L.S.
   1980   "Sex Stereotypes and the American Physician." *Psychology of Women Quarterly* 4, no. 3.

Finn, E.
   1983   *MediCare on the Critical List*. Ottawa: Canadian Centre for Policy Alternatives.

Fisher, S. and S. Groce
   1985   "Doctor-Patient Negotiations of Cultural Assumptions." *Sociology of Health and Illness* 7, no. 3.

Fisher, S. and A. Todd (eds.)
   1986   *Discourse and Institutional Authority*. Norwood, N.J.: Ablex.

Fitzpatrick, R.M.
   1982   "Social Concepts of Disease and Illness." In D.L. Patrick and G. Scambler (eds.), *Sociology as Applied to Medicine*. London: Bailliere Tindall.

Fitzpatrick, R.M. et al.
   1984   *The Experience of Illness*. London: Tavistock.

Flexner, A.
   1972   *Medicine and Society in America*. New York: Arno Press.

Fraser, R.
   1975   *A Research Agenda in Health Care Economics*. Toronto: Ontario Economic Council.

Freudenberg, N.
   1985   "Health Education and the Politics of AIDS." *Health/Pac Bulletin* 16, no. 3.

Friedson, E.
   1966   "Health Factories, The New Industrial Sociology." *Social*
   -67   *Problems* 14.

Friedson, E.
   1970   *Profession of Medicine."* New York: Harper and Row.

Friedson, E.
   1986   "Professional Dominance and the Ordering of Health Services: Some Consequences." In P. Conrad and R. Kern (eds.),

The Sociology of Health and Illness, 2nd ed. New York: St. Martin's Press.

Fry, J.A. (ed.)
1979   *Economy, Class and Social Reality.* Toronto: Butterworths.

Fry, J.A. (ed.)
1984   *Contradictions in Canadian Society.* Toronto: Wiley and Sons.

Garrett, T.
1988   "Women in Medicine." *The New Statesman and Society*, 10 June, p. 30.

Ghan, L. and D. Road
1971   "Relationships Among the Health Team: A Group Practice Reports Its Findings." *Canadian Family Physician* 17, no. 11.

Giddens, A.
1971   *Capitalism and Modern Social Theory.* Cambridge: Cambridge University Press.

Giddens, A.
1982   *Sociology: A Brief But Critical Introduction.* Toronto: Harcourt Brace Jovanovich.

Giesbrecht, E. and J. Brown
1977   *Alcohol Problem in Northwestern Ontario.* Toronto: Addiction Research Foundation.

The Globe and Mail
1987a   "Some Patients Still Face Hefty Changes Despite Ontario Ban on Extra-Billing." 11 February.

The Globe and Mail
1987b   "Cesarean Births Highest in the U.S." Toronto, 12 February.

The Globe and Mail
1987c   "Doctor Faces Hearing Over Valium Treatment." 18 April.

The Globe and Mail
1987d   "Decline in Patient-MD Goodwill Cited as Malpractice Suits Rise." Toronto, 29 May.

Godfrey, M.
1978   "Job Satisfaction – Or Should That Be Dissatisfaction." *Nursing 78*, April and May.

Goffman, E.
1963   *Stigma.* Englewood Cliffs, N.J.: Prentice-Hall

Goleman, D.
1986   "Meaningful Activities and Temperament Key in Satisfaction with Life." *New York Times*, 23 December.

Golub, M.
1985   "Saving Money Losing Lives." *Health/Pac Bulletin* 16, no. 5.

Goode, W.
1960   "Encroachment, Charlatanism and the Emerging Profession: Psychology, Sociology and Medicine." *American Sociological Review* 25, no. b.

Gould, S.J.
1977   *Ever Since Darwin*. New York: W.W. Norton.

Gould, S.J.
1981   *The Mismeasure of Man*. New York: W.W. Norton.

Gould, S.J.
1985   *The Flamingo's Smile*. New York: W.W. Norton.

Graham, H. and A. Oakley
1976   "Competing Ideologies of Reproduction: Medical and Maternal Perspectives on Pregnancy." In Roberts (ed.), *Women, Health and Reproduction*. London: Routledge and Kegan Paul.

Gray-Toft, P. and J. Anderson
1981   "Stress Among Hospital Nursing Staff: Its Cause and Effects." *Social Science and Medicine* 15A, no. 5.

Grayson, J.P.
1985   "The Closure of a Factory and Its Impact on Health." *International Journal of Health Services* 15, no. 1.

Green, F.
1987   "Depo Provera in Canada: Will the Tragedies Ever Stop." *Session* 1, no. 2.

Grescoe, P.
1981   "A Nation's Disgrace." In Coburn et al., *Health and Canadian Society*, 1st ed. Toronto: Fitzhenry and Whiteside.

Hagey, R.
1984   "The Phenomenon, The Explanations and The Responses: Metaphors Surrounding Diabetes in Urban Canadian Indians." *Social Science and Medicine* 18, no. 3.

Haley, B.
1978   *The Healthy Body and Victorian Culture*. Cambridge, Mass.: Harvard University Press.

Hamilton, D.
1987   "Lister and the Surgical Revolution." Lecture presented to the History of Medicine Club, Winnipeg.

Hamowy, R.
1984   *Canadian Medicine: A Study in Restricted Entry*. Toronto: The Fraser Institute.

Hancock, T.
1986   "A Need to Erase the Doctors' Empire." *Winnipeg Free Press*, 21 April.

Hansluwka, H.E.
1985 "Measuring the Health of Populations, Indicators and Interpretations." *Social Science and Medicine* 20, no. 12.

Haralambos, M.
1980 *Sociology: Themes and Perspectives*. London: University Tutorial Press.

Hardin, G.
1985 "Crisis on the Commons." *The Sciences*, September/October.

Harris, L.
1978 *Hospital Care in America*. Poll conducted for Hospital Affiliates International, Nashville.

Hart, N.
1985 *The Sociology of Health and Medicine*. Ormskirk, Britain: Causeway Books.

Hass, J. and W. Shaffir
1978 "The Professionalization of Medical Students." *Symbolic Interaction* 1, no. 1.

Haupt, J. and T. Kane
1985 *Population Handbook*. Washington: Population Reference Bureau.

Heatherington, R.
1986 "Merrijoy Kelner and Peter Kong-New, eds., *Social Science and Health Care in Canada*." *Canadian Journal of Sociology* 11, no. 1.

Health Education Unit, WHO
1986 "Life-Styles and Health." *Social Science and Medicine* 22, no. 2.

Heggenhougen, H.K. and L. Shore
1986 "Cultural Concepts of Behavioural Epidemiology: Implications for Primary Health Care." *Social Science and Medicine* 22, no. 11.

Helman, C.
1984 *Culture, Health and Illness*. Bristol: John Wright and Sons.

Henriques, J. et al.
1984 *Changing the Subject*. New York: Methuen.

Herzlich, C. and J. Pierret
1985 "The Social Construction of the Patient: Patients and Illnesses in Other Ages." *Social Science and Medicine* 20, no. 2.

Hiller, H.M.
1986 *Canadian Society: A Macro Analysis*. Toronto: Prentice-Hall.

Hillier, S.M.
1982a "Medicine and Social Control." In D.L. Patrick and G. Scambler (eds.), *Sociology as Applied to Medicine*. London: Bailliere Tindall.

Hillier, S.M.
 1982b "Women as Patients and Providers." In D.L. Patrick and G. Scambler (eds.), *Sociology as Applied to Medicine*. London: Bailliere Tindall.

Himsworth, H.
 1984 "Epidemiology, Genetics and Sociology." *Journal of Biosocial Science* 16, no. 2.

Hirst, P. and P. Woolley
 1982 *Social Relations and Human Attributes*. London: Tavistock Publications.

Hofling, C. et al.
 1966 "An Experimental Study in Nurse-Physician Relationships." *Journal of Nervous and Mental Disease* 143, no. 2.

Hollingsworth, T.H.
 1969 *Historical Demography*. Cambridge: Cambridge University Press.

Horn, J.
 1969 *Away With All Pests*. New York: Monthly Review Press.

House, J.S.
 1974 "Occupational Stress and Coronary Heart Disease: A Review and Theoretical Integration." *Journal of Health and Social Behaviour* 15, March.

Howell, M.C.
 1978 "Pediatricians and Mothers." In J. Ehrenreich (ed.), *The Cultural Crisis of Modern Medicine*. New York: Monthly Review Press.

Hudelson, E.
 1977 "Mechanical Ventilation from the Patient's Point of View." *Respiratory Care* 22, no. 6.

Hudson, A., G. Hunter, and J. Waddell
 1979 "Iatrogenic Femoral Nerve Injuries." *Canadian Journal of Surgery* 22, no. 1.

Hudson, R.
 1978 "Abraham Flexner in Perspective." In J. Leavitt and R. Numbers (eds.), *Sickness and Health in America*. Madison: University of Wisconsin Press.

Hunter, A.
 1986 *Class Tells: Social Inequality in Canada*. Toronto: Butterworths.

Hurlburt, J.
 1981 "Midwifery in Canada: A Capsule History." *Canadian Nurse* 77, no. 2.

Illich, I.
1976   *Limits to Medicine*. London: Penguin Books.

Innes, J.M.
1977   "Does the Professional Know What the Client Wants?" *Social Science and Medicine* 11, no. 13.

Jaco, E.G. (ed.)
1979   *Patients, Physicians and Illness*. New York: Free Press.

Jager, M.
1982   "Three-Day Strike Action Starts Monday." *Winnipeg Free Press*. 20 November. P. 20.

Jager, M.
1987   "Patients Reminded They Do Have Rights." *Winnipeg Free Press*. April 14.

Jarvis, G. and M. Bolt
1982   "Death Styles Among Canada's Indians." *Social Science and Medicine* 16, no. 14.

Jenkins, K.
1987   "Overusing Respirator Weakens Infants' Muscles." *Medical Post* 23, no. 15.

Johnson, T.
1972   *Professions and Power*. London: Macmillan.

Jones, R.K. and P.A. Jones
1975   *Sociology in Medicine*. Great Britain: The English Universities Press Ltd.

Jordan, B.
1983   *Birth in Four Cultures*. Montreal: Eden Press.

Kaufert, J.M. and W.W. Koolage
1984   "Role Conflict among 'Culture Brokers': The Experience of Native Canadian Medical Interpreters." *Social Science and Medicine* 18, no. 3.

Kaufert, P.
1984   "Women and Their Health in the Middle Years: A Manitoba Project." *Social Science and Medicine* 18, no. 1.

Kelman, S.
1975   "The Social Nature of the Definition Problem in Health." *International Journal of Health Services* 5, no. 4.

Kelner, M. and P. New
1984   "Social Science and Health Care in Canada." *Social Science and Medicine* 18, no. 3.

Kett, J.
1968   *The Formation of the American Medical Profession*. New Haven: Yale University Press.

King, L.
1982 *Medical Thinking: A Historical Preface.* Princeton: Princeton University Press.

Kinnersly, P.
1973 *The Hazards of Work: How to Fight Them.* London: Pluto Press.

Kitcher, P.
1985 *Vaulting Ambition: Sociobiology and the Quest for Human Nature.* Cambridge, Mass.: MIT Press.

Kleinman, A., L. Eisenberg, and B. Good
1978 "Clinical Lessons from Anthropologic and Cross-Cultural Research." *Annals of Internal Medicine* 88, no. 2.

Koran, L.
1975 "The Reliability of Clinical Methods, Data and Judgments." Parts 1 and 2. *New England Journal of Medicine* 293, nos. 13 and 14.

Korcok, M.
1983 "The Ontario Hospital Experiment: American Managers March In." *Canadian Medical Association Journal* 128, no. 6.

Korcok, M.
1985 "The Business of Hearts." *Canadian Medical Association Journal* 132, no. 6.

Kramer, E.A.
1977 *Power and Illness.* New York: Elsevier.

Kuhn, T.
1962 *The Structure of Scientific Revolutions.* Chicago: University of Chicago Press.

Kurtz, M.E., S.M. Johnson, T. Tomlinson, and N.J. Fiel
1985 "Teaching Medical Students the Effects of Values and Stereotyping in the Doctor-Patient Relationship." *Social Science and Medicine* 21, no. 9.

Kurtz, R.A. and H.P. Chalfant
1984 *The Sociology of Medicine.* Toronto: Allyn and Bacon.

Lalonde, M.
1974 *A New Perspective on the Health of Canadians.* Ottawa: Minister
1981 of Supply and Services.

Land, T.
1987 "WHO's Attack on Drug Abuse Begins with Physicians." *Medical Post* 23, no. 15.

Landy, D. (ed.)
1977 *Culture, Disease and Healing.* New York: Macmillan.

Lapierre, L.
1984 *Canadian Women: Profile of Their Health*. Ottawa: Statistics Canada.

Larson, M.
1977 *The Rise of Professionalism*. Berkeley: University of California Press.

Last, J.M.
1982 "Inequalities in Health." Editorial. *Canadian Journal of Public Health* 73, no. 6.

Laws, P.
1977 *X-Rays: More Harm Than Good*. New York: Rodal Press.

Leavitt, J.W.
1986 *Brought to Bed: Childbearing in America, 1750-1950*. Oxford: Oxford University Press.

LeClair, M.
1975 "The Canadian Health Care System." In S. Andreopoulos (ed.), *National Health Insurance*. New York: Wiley.

Lee, Kwang-Sun, L. Gartner, N. Paneth, and L. Tyler
1982 "Recent Trends in Neonatal Mortality: The Canadian Experience." *Canadian Medical Association Journal* 126, no. 4.

Lefebvre, L.A. et al.
1979 *A Prognosis for Hospitals*. Ottawa: Statistics Canada.

Légaré, J. and L. Normandeau-Desjardins
1975 "Infant and Child Mortality among Canadian Eskimos." *Canadian Studies in Population* 2.

LeTouze, D.
1984 "Canada's Health System: Future Trends and Prospects." *Dimensions in Health Care* 16, no. 1.

Levinson, R.
1976 "Sexism in Medicine." *American Journal of Nursing* 76, no. 3.

Levitt, J.
1977 "Men and Women as Providers of Health Care." *Social Science and Medicine* 11, no. 6/7.

Lexchin, J.
1984 *The Real Pushers*. Vancouver: New Star Books.

Lexchin, L.
1987 "Pharmaceutical Promotion in Canada: Convince Them or Confuse Them." *International Journal of Health Services* 17, no. 1.

Lieban, R.
1977   "The Field of Medical Anthropology." In D. Landy (ed.), *Culture, Disease and Healing*. New York: Macmillan.

Light, L. and N. Kleiber
1978   "Interactive Research in a Health Care Setting." *Social Science and Medicine* 12, no. 4A.

Liska, A.E.
1981   *Perspectives on Deviance*. Englewood Cliffs, N.J.: Prentice-Hall.

Losos, J. and M. Trotman
1984   "Estimated Economic Burden of Nosocomial Infection." *Canadian Journal of Public Health* 75, no. 3.

Love, R. and I. Kalnins
1984   "Individualist and Structuralist Perspectives on Nutrition Education for Canadian Children." *Social Science and Medicine* 18, no. 3.

Macfarlane, A.
1984   "A Time to Die?" *International Journal of Epidemiology* 13, no. 1.

Mahood, M.
1973   "Steadily Expanding Medical Service." *Canadian Medical Association Journal* 109, October.

Manitoba
1975   *Vital Statistics*. Winnipeg: Manitoba Department of Health and Social Development.

Manitoba
1983-   *Manitoba, Annual Statistics: 1983-1984*. Winnipeg: Manitoba
84   Health Services Commission.

Manitoba
1985   *Manitoba, Annual Report: Manitoba Health*. Winnipeg: Manitoba Minister of Health.

Mansfield, P.K.
1986   "Like a Boxer Over the Hill?" *Health / Pac Bulletin* 16, no. 6.

Marsden, L.
1974   "Power Within the Medical Profession: Changes in Ontario." Unpublished Paper, University of Toronto.

Marsden, L.
1977   "Power Within a Profession: Medicine in Ontario." *Sociology of Work and Occupations* 4, no. 1.

Martin, M., S. Moyyen, and M. Gelfand
1982   "Cesarean Section: Recent Trends." *The Canadian Journal of Surgery* 25, no. 1.

Mausner, J.S. and S. Kramer
  1985 *Epidemiology: An Introductory Text.* Toronto: W.B. Saunders.

McCormack, T.
  1981 "The New Criticism and the Sick Role." *The Canadian Review of Sociology and Anthropology* 18, no. 1.

McDaniel, S.A.
  1986 *Canada's Aging Population.* Toronto: Butterworths.

McDonnell, K.
  1986 *Adverse Effects: Women and the Pharmaceutical Industry.* Toronto: Women's Press.

McDonnell, K. and M. Valverde
  1985 *The Healthsharing Book.* Toronto: Women's Press.

McGrew, R.F.
  1985 *Encyclopedia of Medical History.* London: Macmillan Press.

McInnes, C.
  1987a "Recognition of Family Practice Increasing." *The Globe and Mail*, Toronto, 6 April.

McInnes, C.
  1987b "An Intern's Life: Battling Exhaustion." *The Globe and Mail*, Toronto, 5 December.

McKeown, T.
  1976 *The Modern Rise of Population.* London: Edward Arnold.

McKeown, T.
  1979 *The Role of Medicine.* Princeton: Princeton University Press.

McKinley, J.B.
  1981 "A Case for Refocussing Upstream: The Political Economy of Illness." In P. Conrad and R. Kern (eds.), *The Sociology of Health and Illness*, 1st ed. New York: St. Martin's Press.

McKinley, J.B. (ed.)
  1981 *Health Maintenance Organizations.* Milbank Reader No. 5. Cambridge, Mass.: MIT Press.

McKinley, J.B. (ed.)
  1984 *Issues in the Political Economy of Health Care.* London: Tavistock.

McKinley, P.
  1987 "Pilot Project to Pay Doctors Flat Patient Fee." *Winnipeg Free Press*, 7 April.

McLachlan, G. and T. McKeown (eds.)
  1971 *Medical History and Medical Care.* London: Oxford University Press.

McMonagale, D.
  1986   "Ontario MDs Set Strike to Protect Extra-Billing." *The Globe and Mail*, Toronto, 23 May.

McNevin, S., P. Leichner, D. Harper, and E. McCrimmon
  1985   "Sex Role Ideology Among Health Care Professionals." *The Psychiatric Journal of The University of Ottawa* 10, no. 1.

McPhee, J.
  1974   "Further Discussion on Saskatchewan CHA Clinics Evaluation." *Canadian Medical Association Journal* 110, no. 2.

McPherson, K., P. Strong, A. Epstein, and L. Jones
  1981   "Regional Variations in the Use of Common Surgical Procedures: Within and Between England and Wales, Canada and the United States." *Social Science and Medicine* 15, no. 1.

McQuaig, L.
  1986   "Doctors Carry On." *This Magazine* 20, no. 1.

Mechanic, D.
  1978   *Medical Sociology*, 2nd ed. New York: The Free Press.

Menzies, R.J.
  1985   "Genetic Ideology: Observations on the Biologicization of Sociology." *The Canadian Review of Sociology and Anthropology* 22, no. 2.

Michaels, E.
  1982   "The HSO Experiment: Better Than Fee-For-Service?" *Canadian Medical Association Journal* 127, no. 5.

Migue, J.-L. and G. Belenger
  1974   *The Price of Health*. Toronto: Macmillan.

Milio, N.
  1975   "Values, Social Class and Community Health Services." In C. Cox and A. Mead (eds.), *A Sociology of Medical Practice*. London: Collier-Macmillan.

Millman, M.
  1977   *The Unkindest Cut*. New York: William Morrow.

Millman, M.
  1986   "Medical Mortality Review: A Cordial Affair." In P. Conrad and R. Kern (eds.), *The Sociology of Health and Illness*. New York: St. Martin's Press.

Mills, C.W.
  1959   *The Sociological Imagination*. London: Oxford University Press.

Mishler, E.G.
  1981a "The Health-Care System: Social Contexts and Consequences." In E.G. Mishler et al. (eds.), *Social Contexts of Health*,

Illness and Patient Care. Cambridge: Cambridge University Press.

Mishler, E.G.
  1981b   "The Social Construction of Illness." In E.G. Mishler et al. (eds.), *Social Contexts of Health, Illness and Patient Care.* Cambridge: Cambridge University Press.

Mishler, E.G.
  1984   *The Discourse of Medicine.* Norwood, N.J.: Ablex Publishing.

Mishler, E.G. et al. (eds.)
  1981   *Social Contexts of Health, Illness and Patient Care.* Cambridge: Cambridge University Press.

Moccia, P.
  1982   "The Case of the Missing Nurse." *Health/Pac Bulletin* 13, no. 5.

Moore, T.
  1985   "Patients Are Not Consumers." *Winnipeg Free Press*, 13 February.

Morgan, M., M. Calnan, and N. Manning
  1985   *Sociological Approaches to Health and Medicine.* London: Croom Helm.

Moser, R.H.
  1956   "Diseases of Medical Progress." *The New England Journal of Medicine* 255, no. 13.

Moulton, D.
  1987   "Health Costs Blamed for Nova Scotia's Large Debt." *Medical Post* 23, no. 15.

Muller, C.
  1986   "Women and Men: Quality and Equality in Health Care." *Social Policy* 17.

Mumford, E.
  1983   *Medical Sociology.* Toronto: Random House.

Murray, V., T. Jick, and P. Bradshaw
  1984   "Hospital Funding Constraints: Strategic and Tactical Decision Responses to Sustained Moderate Levels of Crisis in Six Canadian Hospitals." *Social Science and Medicine* 18, no. 3.

Myer, J.H.
  1983   "Midwifery: An International Perspective." *Journal of Nurse-Midwifery* 28, no. 5.

Nathanson, C.A.
  1978   "Illness and the Feminine Role: A Theoretical Review." In H.D. Schwartz and C.S. Kart (eds.), *Dominant Issues in Medical Sociology.* Don Mills, Ontario: Addison-Wesley.

Navarro, V.
1976   *Medicine Under Capitalism*. New York: Prodist Press.

Navarro, V.
1977   *Health and Medical Care in the U.S.: A Critical Analysis*. New York: Baywood Publishing.

Naylor, C.D.
1986   *Private Practice, Public Payment*. Kingston: McGill-Queen's University Press.

Normandeau, L. and J. Légaré
1979   "La mortalité infantile des Inuit du Nouveau-Quebec." *The Canadian Review of Sociology and Anthropology* 16, no. 3.

Northcott, H.
1980   "Women, Work and Health." *Pacific Sociological Review* 23, no. 4.

Novak, M.
1985   *Successful Aging*. Toronto: Penguin Books.

Oakley, A.
1980   *Women Confined: Towards a Sociology of Childbirth*. Oxford: Martin Robinson.

Oakley, A.
1984   *The Captured Womb*. New York: Basil Blackwell.

Oakley, A.
1987   "From Walking Wombs to Test-Tube Babies." In M. Stanworth (ed.), *Reproductive Technologies*. Oxford: Polity Press.

Oglov, L.
1985   "Mall Medicine – Convenient, But What About the Quality of Care." *Canadian Medical Association Journal* 132, no. 4.

Ohlsson, A. and L. Fohlin
1983   "Reproductive Medical Care in Sweden and the Province of Ontario, Canada." *Acta Paediatrica Scandinavica*, Supplement 306.

O'Neill, J.
1986   "The Medicalization of Social Control." *The Canadian Review of Sociology and Anthropology* 23, no. 3.

Overbeek, J.
1980   *Population and Canadian Society*. Toronto: Butterworths.

Owens, A.
1983   "Who Says Doctors Make Too Much Money." *Medical Economics*, 7 March.

Pablo, R. and F. Cleary
   1982   "Parkwood Day Hospital: An Alternative for the Impaired Elderly." *Canadian Journal of Public Health* 73, no. 3.

Parlow, J. and A.I. Rothman
   1974   "Personality traits of first year medical students: trends over a six year period, 1967-1972." *British Journal of Medical Education* 8, no. 1.

Parsons, T.
   1951   "Illness and the Role of the Physician." In Kluckhohn, Murray and Schneider, *Personality in Nature, Culture and Society.* New York: Knopf.

Parsons, T.
   1953   *The Social System.* New York: The Free Press.

Patrick, D.L. and G. Scambler (eds.)
   1982   *Sociology as Applied to Medicine.* London: Bailliere Tindall.

Pearce, J.
   1985   "Ultrasound in Obstetrics." *The Practitioner* 229, August.

Pendleton, D.A. and S. Bochner
   1980   "The Communication of Medical Information in General Practice Consultations as a Function of Patients' Social Class." *Social Science and Medicine* 14A, no. 6.

Peron, Y. and C. Strohmenger
   1985   *Demographic and Health Indicators.* Ottawa: Statistics Canada.

Postl, B.
   1975   "Gas Sniffing in Shamattawa." *University of Manitoba Medical Journal* 45, no. 3.

Powis, J.
   1981   "The Quiet Revolution: Establishing a Nurse-Midwifery Practice." *Canadian Nurse* 77, no. 2.

Price, R.A. and W. McCormick
   1981   "The Declining Autopsy Rate and Its Significance for Neuropathology: Two Viewpoints." *Journal of Neuropathology and Experimental Neurology* 40, no. 5.

Prior, L.
   1985   "Making Sense of Mortality." *Sociology of Health and Illness* 7, no. 2.

Randall, C.
   1980   "The Problem of Pseudomonas cepacia in a Hospital." *Canadian Journal of Public Health* 71, no. 2.

Ray, A.J.
   1981   "Diffusion of Disease in the Western Interior of Canada." In
          S.E.D. Shortt (ed.), *Medicine in Canadian Society*. Montreal:
          McGill-Queen's University Press.

Reading, A.
   1977   "Illness and Disease." *Medical Clinics of North America* 61, no. 4.

Reasons, C., L. Ross, and C. Paterson
   1981   *Assault on the Worker*. Toronto: Butterworths.

Reeder, S.J. and H. Mauksch
   1979   "Nursing: Continuing Change." In H. Freeman, S. Levine
          and L. Reeder (eds.), *Handbook of Medical Sociology*, 3rd ed.
          Toronto: Prentice-Hall.

Reiker, P. and J. Begun
   1980   "Translating Social Science Concepts into Medical Education:
          A Model and a Curriculum." *Social Science and Medicine* 14a,
          no. 6.

Reiser, S.J.
   1978   *Medicine and the Reign of Technology*. Cambridge: Cambridge
          University Press.

Renaud, M.
   1978   "On the Structural Constraints of State Intervention." In J.
          Ehrenreich (ed.), *The Cultural Crisis of Modern Medicine*. New
          York: Monthly Review Press.

Rich, P.
   1987   "Ontario Will Review Funding System for Hospitals." *Medical
          Post* 23, no. 15.

Riffel, J.A, J. Burelle, and J.P. Kelly
   1972   *The Quality of Life of Native Peoples*. Winnipeg: University of
          Manitoba.

Rinehart, J.
   1975   *The Tyranny of Work*. Toronto: Academic Press Canada.

Roedde, G.
   1979   "Health Care for Indians." *Canadian Medical Association Jour-
          nal* 121, November.

Roemer, M.
   1981   "More Data on the Post-Surgical Deaths Related to the Los
          Angeles Doctor Slowdown." *Social Science and Medicine* 15c,
          no. 3.

Roemer, M. and J. Schwartz
   1979   "Doctor Slowdown: Effects on the Population of Los Angeles
          County." *Social Science and Medicine* 13c, no. 4.

Rombout, M.K.
  1975 *Health Care Institutions and Canada's Elderly: 1971-2031.* Ottawa: Health and Welfare Canada.

Rose, G. and D.J.P. Barker
  1979 *Epidemiology for the Uninitiated.* London: British Medical Association.

Rose, S. et al. (eds.)
  1985a *Medical Knowledge: Doubt and Certainty.* London: Open University Press.

Rose, S. et al. (eds.)
  1985b *Studying Health and Disease.* London: Open University Press.

Rosedale, M.
  1965 "Health in a Sick Society." *New Left Review* no. 34.

Roth, J.
  1985 "Consistency of Rule Application to Inmates in Long-Term Treatment Institutions." *Social Science and Medicine* 20, no. 3.

Roth, J. and S. Ruzek (eds.)
  1986 *Research in the Sociology of Health Care: The Adoption and Social Consequences of Medical Technology.* London: Jai Press.

Rothman, B. Katz
  1983 "Midwives in Transition: The Structure of a Clinical Revolution: The Structure of a Clinical Revolution." *Social Problems* 30, no. 3.

Rowe, G. and M.J. Norris
  1985 *Mortality Projections on Registered Indians.* Ottawa: Indian and Northern Affairs.

Rowland, A.J. and P. Cooper
  1983 *Environment and Health.* London: Edward Arnold.

Rozovsky, L.E.
  1979 *Canadian Hospital Law*, 2nd ed. Ottawa: Canadian Hospital Association.

Rozovsky, L.E.
  1980 *The Canadian Patient's Book of Rights.* Toronto: Doubleday.

Ruderman, A.P.
  1974 "The Drug Business in the Context of Canadian Health Care Programs." *International Journal of Health Services* 4, no. 4.

Ryder, N.
  1964 "Notes on the Concept of Population." *American Journal of Sociology* 69, no. 5.

Ryten, E. and M. Watanabe
  1987   "A Diagnosis of Doctor Glut Raises Doubt." *The Globe and Mail*, Toronto, 19 May.

Sahlins, M.
  1977   *The Use and Abuse of Biology*. London: Tavistock.

Sanazaro, P.
  1971   "Historical Discontinuity, Hospitals, and Health Services." In G. McLachlan and T. McKeown (eds.), *Medical History and Medical Care*. London: Oxford University Press.

Sand, R.
  1952   *The Advance to Social Medicine*. London: Staples Press.

Sass, R.
  1980   "Dying for a Living." *Canadian Dimension* 14, no. 7.

Schaefer, O.
  1973   "The Changing Health Picture in the Canadian North." *Canadian Journal of Opthalmology*. 8, no. 1.

Schwartz, H. and C. Kart (eds.)
  1978   *Dominant Issues in Medical Sociology*. Toronto: Addison-Wesley.

Scully, D. and P. Bart
  1978   "A Funny Thing Happened on the Way to the Orifice: Women in Gynecology Textbooks." In J. Ehrenreich (ed.), *The Cultural Crisis of Modern Medicine*. New York: Monthly Review Press.

Segall, A.
  1976   "The Sick Role Concept: Understanding Illness Behaviour." *Journal of Health and Social Behaviour* 17, no. 1.

Segall, A. and M. Burnett
  1980   "Patient Evaluation of Physician Role Performance." *Social Science and Medicine* 14A, no. 4.

Segall, A. and R. Currie
  1983   "Selected Findings from the 1983 Winnipeg Area Study." Series Report No. 1. Winnipeg: Institute for Social and Economic Research, University of Manitoba.

Sennett, R. and J. Cobb
  1972   *The Hidden Injuries of Class*. New York: Vintage Books.

Sevely, J. Lowndes
  1987   *Eve's Secrets: A New Perspective on Human Sexuality*. London: Bloomsbury.

Shalom, F.
  1987   "Quebec Doctors' Group Recommends User-Fees." *The Globe and Mail*, Toronto, 28 April.

Shapiro, M.
   1978   *Getting Doctored: Critical Reflections on Becoming a Physician.* Kitchener: Between the Lines.

Shepard, A.E.
   1976   "Methylmercury Poisoning in Canada." *Canadian Medical Association Journal* 114, no. 15.

Shortt, S.E.D. (ed.)
   1981   *Medicine in Canadian Society: Historical Perspectives.* Montreal: McGill-Queen's University Press.

Showalter, E.
   1985   *The Female Malady.* New York: Pantheon Books.

Sidel, V. and R. Sidel
   1984   *Reforming Medicine.* New York: Pantheon.

Silver, J.
   1984   "The Erosion of Medicare." *Canadian Dimension* 18, no. 2.

Silversides, A.
   1987a   "Court Upholds B.C. Control on the Supply, Location of MDs." *The Globe and Mail*, Toronto, 7 January.

Silversides, A.
   1987b   "Wealthy Face Shorter Wait For Chronic Care Beds, Experts Say." *The Globe and Mail*, Toronto, 21 April.

Silversides, A.
   1987c   "Revamp Hospital Financing, Study Urges." *The Globe and Mail*, Toronto, 23 April.

Silversides, A.
   1987d   "Some Patients Still Face Hefty Charges Despite Ontario Ban on Extra-Billing." *The Globe and Mail*, Toronto, 11 February.

Singh Bolaria, B.
   1979   "Self-Care and Lifestyles: Ideological and Policy Implications." In J.A. Fry (ed.), *Economy, Class and Social Reality.* Toronto: Butterworths.

Sisk, J., C. Behney, and H. Banta
   1984   "Evaluating the Costs of Medical Technology." *Research in the Sociology of Health Care* 3.

Skelton, D.
   1982   "The Hospice Movement: A Human Approach to Palliative Care." *Canadian Medical Association Journal* 126, no. 5.

Skipper, J. and R. Leonard
   1965   *Social Interaction and Patient Care.* Montreal: J.B. Lippincott.

Smith, J.
   1984   "Slow Death of the Autopsy." *Human Pathology* 15, no. 2.

Snider, E.
1980 "The Elderly and their Doctors." *Social Science and Medicine* 14A, no. 6.

Sobel, D. (ed.)
1979 *Ways of Health: Holistic Approaches to Ancient and Contemporary Medicine.* New York: Harcourt Brace Jovanovich.

Soderstrom, L.
1978 *The Canadian Health System.* London: Croom Helm.

Soderstrom, L.
1982 *Taxing the Sick.* Ottawa: Canadian Centre for Policy Alternatives.

Soderstrom, L.
1986 "Effects of Unemployment on the Health of Unemployed Married Women." Paper presented at Third Canadian Conference on Health Economics, Winnipeg.

Speirs, D.
1986 "VDT Safety Doubted by Labour." *Winnipeg Free Press*, 16 August.

Spradlin, W.W. and P.B. Porterfield
1979 *Human Biosociology.* New York: Springer-Verlag.

Stanworth, M. (ed.)
1987 *Reproductive Technologies: Gender, Motherhood and Medicine.* Oxford: Polity Press.

Starr, P.
1982 *The Social Transformation of American Medicine.* New York: Basic Books.

Staum, M. and D. Larsen (eds.)
1981 *Doctors, Patients and Society.* Waterloo: Wilfrid Laurier Press.

Steel, K., P. Gertman, C. Crescenzi, and J. Anderson
1981 "Iatrogenic Illness on a General Medical Service at a University Hospital." *The New England Journal of Medicine* 304, no. 11.

Stein, L.I.
1967 "The Doctor-Nurse Game." *Archives of General Psychiatry* 16, June.

Stektasa, R.
1977 "Health Care in Canada." *The Financial Post*, 1 January.

Stoddart, G. and R. Labelle
1985 *Privatization in the Canadian Health Care System.* Ottawa: Minister of National Health and Welfare.

Strauss, A.
1975 "A Sociologist's Perspective." In J. Howard and A. Strauss (eds.), *Humanizing Health Care*. New York: Wiley and Sons.

Strauss, R.
1957 "The Nature and Status of Medical Sociology." *American Sociological Review* 22, no. 2.

Stroman, D.
1976 *The Medical Establishment and Social Responsibility*. New York: Kennikat Press.

Suleiman, S.R. (ed.)
1986 *The Female Body in Western Culture*. Cambridge, Mass.: Harvard University Press.

Susser, M., W. Watson, and K. Hopper
1985 *Sociology in Medicine*. Oxford: Oxford University Press.

Sutherland, M.
1976 "Mercury Pollution." *University of Manitoba Medical Journal* 46, no. 4.

Swartz, M.
1977 "The Politics of Reform: Conflict and Accommodation in Canadian Health Policy." In L. Panitch (ed.), *The Canadian State*. Toronto: University of Toronto Press.

Syme, S. and L. Berkman
1986 "Social Class, Susceptibility and Sickness." In P. Conrad and R. Kern (eds.), *The Sociology of Health and Illness*, 2nd ed. New York: St. Martin's Press.

Szasz, T. and M. Hollender
1956 "The Basic Models of the Doctor-Patient Relationship." *Archives in Internal Medicine* 97, no. 5.

Taylor, K.M.
1988 " 'Telling bad news': Physicians and the Disclosure of Undesirable Information." *Sociology of Health and Illness* 10, no. 2.

Taylor, M.G., H.M. Stevenson, and A.P. Williams
1984 "Medical Perspectives on Canadian Medicare: Attitudes of Canadian Physicians to Policies and Problems of the Medical Care Insurance Program." Institute for Behavioural Research, York University, Toronto.

Thomas, J. (ed.)
1983 *Medical Ethnics and Human Life*. Toronto: Samuel Stevens.

Thomas, L.
1983 "On the AIDS Problem." *Discover* 4.

Thompson, J.
   1984   "Communicating with Patients." In R.M. Fitzpatrick et al. (eds.) *The Experience of Illness*. London: Tavistock.

Topliss, E.
   1978   "Common Concerns in Health Care." In P. Brearley et al., *The Social Context of Health Care*. Oxford: Blackwell and Robertson.

Torrance, G.
   1987   "Socio-Historical Overview." In D. Coburn et al., *Health and Canadian Society*, 2nd ed. Toronto: Fitzhenry and Whiteside.

Totman, R.
   1979   *The Social Causes of Illness*. London: Souvenir Press.

Trowler, P.
   1984   *Topics in Sociology*. Slough: University Tutorial Press.

Tuckett, D. and J. Kaufert (eds.)
   1978   *Basic Readings in Medical Sociology*. London: Tavistock.

Turner, B.S.
   1987   *Medical Power and Social Knowledge*. London: Sage.

Turner, G.P. and J. Mapa
   1981   *The Choice Is Yours*. Toronto: McGraw-Hill Ryerson.

United States
   1985   *Preventing Lead Poisoning in Young Children*. Atlanta: Center for Disease Control.

Van Wart, A.F.
   1948   "The Indians of the Maritime Provinces, Their Diseases and Native Cures." *Canadian Medical Association Journal* 59, no. 6.

Vavasour, M. and Y. Mennie
   ND   "For Health or For Profit?" Health Kit. Ottawa: Inter Pares/ World Inter-Action.

Vayda, E.
   1973   "A Comparison of the Surgical Rates in Canada and in England and Wales." *The New England Journal of Medicine* 289, no. 23 (December).

Vayda, E.
   1978   "Health Policy in Canada: The Lalonde Report and Emerging Patterns." In Carlson and Cunningham (eds.), *Future Directions in Health Care*. Cambridge: Ballinger.

Vayda, E. and R. Deber
   1984   "The Canadian Health Care System: An Overview." *Social Science and Medicine* 18, no. 3.

Vayda, E., W. Mindell, and I. Rutkow
   1982   "A Decade of Surgery in Canada, England and Wales and the U.S." *Archives of Surgery* 117, June.

Veitch, A.
　1986a　"Up to 10 Million Affected by AIDS." *Manchester Guardian Weekly*, 29 June.

Veitch, A.
　1986b　"Class Link Health Gap Grows." *Manchester Guardian Weekly*, 10 August.

Veitch, A.
　1988a　" 'Second Wave' of AIDS Spreads Beyond Risk Groups." *The Guardian*, 9 February.

Veitch, A.
　1988b　"The Cruel March of AIDS." *The Guardian*, 16 February.

Veith, I.
　1965　*Hysteria: The History of a Disease.* Chicago: University of Chicago Press.

Wadhera, S.
　1982　"Trends in Cesarean Section Deliveries, Canada." *Canadian Journal of Public Health* 73, no. 1.

Wahn, M.
　1983　"The Health of the Working Class." *Canadian Dimension* 17, no. 1.

Wahn, M.
　1984a　"Rising Health Costs." *Canadian Dimension* 18, no. 2.

Wahn, M.
　1984b　"Losing Medicare: Why Worry?" *Canadian Dimension* 17, no. 1.

Wahn, M.
　1985　"Research on Nurses' Work in Hospitals: An Annotated Bibliography." Unpublished paper. University of Winnipeg.

Wahn, M.
　1987　"The Decline of Medical Dominance in Hospitals." In D. Coburn et al. (eds.) *Health and Canadian Society*, 2nd ed. Toronto: Fitzhenry and Whiteside.

Waitzkin, H.
　1979　"Medicine, Superstructure and Micropolitics." *Social Science and Medicine* 13A, no. 6.

Waitzkin, H.
　1986　"Micropolitics of Medicine: Theoretical Issues." *Medical Anthropology Quarterly* 17, no. 5.

Waitzkin, H. and J. Stoeckle
　1976　"Information Control and the Micropolitics of Health Care: Summary of an Ongoing Research Project." *Social Science and Medicine* 10, no. 6.

Waldron, I.
  1986   "Why Do Women Live Longer Than Men?" In P. Conrad and
         R. Kern (eds.), *The Sociology of Health and Illness*. New York: St.
         Martin's Press.

Wallace, A.
  1986   "Teaching the Human Touch." *New York Times Magazine*, 28
         December.

Walsh, M.
  1979   "The Rediscovery of Need for a Feminist Medical Educa-
         tion." *Harvard Educational Review* 49, no. 4.

Walters, V.
  1982a "State, Capital and Labour: the Introduction of Federal-
         Provincial Insurance for Physician Care in Canada." *The
         Canadian Review of Sociology and Anthropology* 19, no. 2.

Walters, V.
  1982b "Company Doctors' Perceptions of and Responses to Conflict-
         ing Pressures From Labour and Management." *Social Problems*
         30, no. 1.

Walters, V.
  1983   "Occupational Health and Safety Legislation in Ontario: An
         Analysis of Its Origins and Content." *The Canadian Review of
         Sociology and Anthropology* 20, no. 4.

Walters, V.
  1985   "The Politics of Occupational Health and Safety." *The Cana-
         dian Review of Sociology and Anthropology* 22, no. 1.

Walton, J., P. Beeson, and R.B. Scott
  1986   *The Oxford Companion to Medicine*. 2 Vols. Oxford: Oxford
         University Press.

Warner, K.E.
  1985   "Cigarette Advertising and Media Coverage of Smoking and
         Health." *The New England Journal of Medicine* 312, no. 6.

Weaver, J.L. and S.D. Garrett
  1978   "Sexism and Racism in the American Health Care Industry."
         International Journal of Health Services 8, no. 4.

Weidman, H.
  1981   "Dominance and Domination in Health Care: A Trans-
         Cultural Perspective." In M. Staum and D. Larsen (eds.),
         Doctors, Patients and Society. Waterloo: Wilfrid Laurier Press.

Weller, G.R.
  1977   "From 'Pressure Group Politics' to 'Medical Industrial Com-
         plex': The Development of Approaches to the Politics of
         Health." *Journal of Health Politics, Policy and Law* 1, no. 4.

Weller, G.R. and P. Manga
1983 "The Push for Reprivatization of Health Care Services in Canada, Britain and the United States." *Journal of Health Politics, Policy and Law* 8, no. 3.

Weston, M. and B. Jeffery
1988 "AIDS: The Politicizing of a Public Health Issue." In B. Singh Bolaria and H. Dickinson (eds.), *Sociology of Health Care in Canada*. Toronto: Harcourt Brace Jovanovich.

Wigle, D.T. and Y. Mao
1980 *Mortality by Income Level in Urban Canada*. Ottawa: Minister of National Health and Welfare, Health Protection Branch.

Wilensky, H.
1964 "The Professionalisation of Everyone?" *American Journal of Sociology* 69, September.

Wilkins, R.
1980a "Differential Mortality in Montreal: 1961-1976." Presented at the meetings of the Canadian Population Society, Montreal.

Wilkins, R.
1980b *Health Status in Canada, 1926-1976*. Occasional Paper No. 13. Montreal: Institute for Research on Public Policy.

Wilkins, R. and O.B. Adams
1982 "The Distribution of Health Expectancy in Canada: Demographic, Regional and Social Dimensions." Paper presented at the Meetings of the CSAA, Ottawa.

Wilkinson, R.G. (ed.)
1986 *Class and Health*. London: Tavistock.

Williams, R.
1980 *Materialism and Culture*. London: New Left Books.

Winnipeg Free Press
1982 "Doctors Need Public Support." 20 November.

Winnipeg Free Press
1983 "MD Blames Access for Doctor Addicts." 27 October.

Winnipeg Free Press
1986a "A House for Dying." 12 August.

Winnipeg Free Press
1986b "Addicted Nurses Blame Stress of Job." 23 July.

Winnipeg Free Press
1986c "Ontario MD Hires Goons, Loses License." 13 December.

Winnipeg Free Press
1986d "AIDS Will Kill Millions, Report Predicts." 26 November.

Winnipeg Free Press
  1986e   "Doctor's Donation Request Irks Woman." 21 January.
Winnipeg Free Press
  1987a   "Medical Fraud Astonishes Court." 21 January.
Winnipeg Free Press
  1987b   "Province Seeks Limit System to Govern Doctors' Fee
          Increase." 21 February.
Wolfe, S.
  1964   "Saskatchewan's Community Clinics." *Canadian Medical Asso-
          ciation Journal* 91, no. 5.
Wolfe, S. and R. Badgley
  1973   *The Family Doctor*. Toronto: Macmillan.
Wolfson, A.D. and C.J. Tuohy
  1980   *Opting Out of Medicare*. Toronto: Published for the Ontario
          Economic Council by University of Toronto Press.
Women's Health Interaction Manitoba
  1987   "Statement of Goals." *Health Network Update*, no. 1. Winnipeg.
Woods, D.
  1983   "The Alleged MD Surplus: A Need for Superb Data, National
          Policy." *Canadian Medical Association Journal* 129, no. 11.
York, G.
  1987a   "Education Not Needed Here, Saskatchewan Says of AIDS."
          The Globe and Mail, Toronto, 4 March.
York, G.
  1987b   "Patients Left Out of Major Decisions, Medical Study Says."
          The Globe and Mail, Toronto, 29 April.
Young, T.K.
  1983   "Mortality Patterns of Isolated Indians in Northwestern
          Ontario: A Ten Year Review." *Public Health Reports* 95, no. 5.
Young, T.K.
  1984   "Indian Health Services in Canada: A Sociohistorical Perspec-
          tive." *Social Science and Medicine* 18, no. 3.
Young, T.K. and N.W. Choi
  1985   "Cancer Risks Among Residents of Manitoba Indian
          Reserves, 1970-1979." *Canadian Medical Association Journal*
          132, no. 11.
Zeitlin, I.
  1984   *The Social Construction of Humanity*. New York: Oxford Univer-
          sity Press.
Zimbardo, P.
  1972   "Pathology of Imprisonment." *Society* 9.

Zinsser, H.
  1935   *Rats, Lice and History.* New York: Blue Ribbon Books.

Zola, I.K.
  1966   "Culture and Symptoms: An Analysis of Patients' Presenting
         Complaints." *American Sociological Review* 31.

Zola, I.K.
  1972   "Medicine as an Institution of Social Control." *The Sociological
         Review* 20, no. 4 (November).

Zola, I.K.
  1973   "Pathways to the Doctor – From Person to Patient." *Social
         Science and Medicine* 7, no. 9.

Zola, I.K.
  1975   "In the Name of Health and Illness: On Some Socio-Political
         Consequences of Medical Influence." *Social Science and Medi-
         cine* 9, no. 2.

Zola, I.K.
  1983   *Socio-Medical Inquiries.* Philadelphia: Temple University Press.

Index

Edginton, Barry

Health, disease and medicine
in Canada: a sociological
perspective